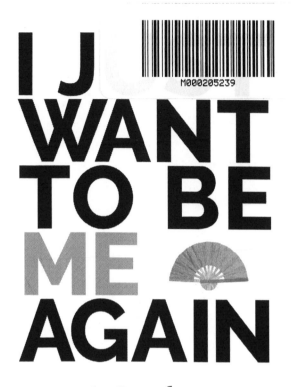

# I WANT TO BE ME AGAIN

## A Guide to Thriving Through Menopause

BY JEANNE D. ANDRUS

THE MENOPAUSE GURU™

difference press

## COPYRIGHT

## DISCLAIMER

*Cover Design*: John Matthews

*Interior Design*: Heidi Miller

*Editing*: Grace Kerina

Author's photo courtesy of Rupa Kapoor, Woman Redefined

# DEDICATION

*To you, my reader.*

*During your menopausal journey, may you find yourself again.*

*And to my strong and daring girlfriends, Karen, Liz, Tara, and Kat.*

*Without your support, I'd have lost my way many more times than I did.*

# TABLE OF CONTENTS

# CHAPTER 1

# ALL I WANTED WAS TO BE ME AGAIN

It was February 14th — Valentine's Day — and I was in the tropical paradise of Belize, which was in love with love. It seemed that the whole country was decorated with cupids and hearts, but all I could do was cry.

I was crying because my life was broken and I just wanted the old me back. The day before, at the marriage counselor's office, my 27-year marriage had been declared brain-dead and the plug had been pulled.

I was between jobs and so had booked a vacation to Belize. My husband and I had had great vacations in Belize in the past, and I'd been disappointed that he'd decided not to come along when I'd planned the trip. It turns out that was a good thing, because the day before I left we decided to "take a break from our marriage".

That Valentine's Day, I didn't know how much I had yet to lose. My marriage was gone, and the house I loved would be next. Before long, my relationship with my college-age son would also be endangered. But I was pretty sure the worst part was that I'd lost myself.

I didn't really know what was going on with me, but I did know I hadn't felt like myself in a very long time. I was

48 years old and, oddly enough, my periods were more regular than they'd ever been, even if my moods and my temper weren't.

So, there I was, on a vacation in paradise, all by myself. It seemed like eating was the thing to do. That was the start of a six-week binge. I stuffed myself with all manner of comfort food as I attempted to get past the feeling of utter failure as I watched my world crumble. By the time six weeks had passed, I'd gained 30 pounds, adding to the extra 50 pounds I already carried.

My self-esteem was gone. My marriage was gone. I was working for a new company and felt completely alone for the first time in a long time. I had committed to selling the home I loved and moving 1800 miles away to move in with my aging mother.

I had no idea who I was anymore, and I really wasn't fond of this person I'd become. I was lost, shaken, and confused, and I just wanted to feel like myself again.

And I had no idea how to do that.

## WHY DIDN'T ANYONE TELL ME ABOUT THIS?

Remember back when you were growing up and, sometime around fourth or fifth grade, the school nurse and one of the teachers (always a woman!) took all the girls into a classroom to show you a movie about (gasp!) menstruation? The boys got to go play basketball and we got to be scared out of our wits!

I remember that we had to have a signed permission slip, which no one's mother *wouldn't* sign, because then she'd be stuck explaining this particular set of the facts of life to her daughter. I suspect the girls with older sisters were already in the know, but my best friends were all either the only girls in their family (like me) or the oldest girls, so we were clueless.

As awful as that moment of revelation was, learning about menstruation that way was a million times better than if I'd been blindsided by a first period with no notion of what it was about. That happened to a few of my friends who attended parochial schools. One of them told me the story of how she hid her panties from her mother for several days, went to confession, and went home to prepare to die. I've forgotten how she actually found out the bleeding was normal, but her fear that she'd been dying was still obvious when she told me this story several years later.

You'd think, after realizing how important it was to know our menstrual cycles would be starting soon, *someone* would've figured out how important it would be to know about them ending.

But, no! No one calls us into a classroom with other 40-year-olds to show us a cute little film that tells us what we're about to go through. Maybe they figure that if we really knew about menopause ahead of time, we might all refuse to continue to do our jobs as wives and mothers and demand that we be given "retirement with full pay."

Well, then, maybe our doctors should warn us. Except that so many of them have no understanding of what's going on, either. Most of the research I've done, both for this book and for work with my clients, was published in this century, and a good deal of it is so new that it's only on the Internet. I recently read a "forward-thinking" book about menopause that was published in 1991 and it doesn't even mention progesterone. That's because, even in 1991, so little was known about it.

Unless a doctor is dedicated to keeping current in the specialty of menopause, they may bring an outdated view into their consultations with you. And it's unlikely that they consider it their job to inform you about what's going on in your body regarding menopause (though they might tell you more than you already know, if you ask them).

Even my gynecologist, who really is one of the good gals, assumed I already knew what was going on with my body and menopause. I sensed her assumption because she couched her questions and advice in language ambiguous enough that I could answer truthfully while still not really knowing that she was talking about menopause.

Maybe our moms should tell us about menopause. Yeah, right. Like that was gonna happen for me. My mom was relieved that my school told me about menstruation. She never explained sex to me and seemed pretty oblivious about pregnancy (in fairness, my brother and I were adopted, so she hadn't experienced it). So menopause was pretty much a lost cause as a topic for discussion. Besides, our moms went through menopause during a time when doctors didn't understand about menopause to a much greater degree than now, so what they did understand was bound to be pretty simplistic.

## THREE MIRACLES

So, there I was, 80 pounds overweight, miserably unhappy, and about to embark on a move to a place I wasn't sure I wanted to live and to work for a company I wasn't sure I wanted to work for. Somewhere, deep inside, there was just one little spark left. Maybe it was a spark of anger, or maybe it was hope. All I know is that spark said, *I can let this kill me, or I can let this be the best thing that ever happened to me.* That spark was my first miracle.

I don't know if I've fully spelled out for myself — before this moment as I write — exactly what the "this" was in what that spark told me. I thought at first that it was about my divorce. But it was about more than that. It included *all of it*, everything about my life — moving home to mama, being 80 pounds overweight, leaving New England and my son, and moving 1800 miles away. My life was changing and I felt uprooted. All of that outside stuff was a reflection of what was going on inside me.

What was going on was perimenopause. The Change of Life. I could let it destroy me, or I could let it be the best thing that ever happened to me.

When that spark said its thing, I decided then and there that all the changes I was going through *were* going to be the best thing that ever happened to me. I knew that almost nothing was in my control at that moment, and that I had to give over control of just about everything to God. But I took control of the one thing I could control: what I put in my mouth, what I ate. (Like many perimenopausal women, I didn't have a whole lot of control over what came out of my mouth!)

The second miracle occurred a few days later. My doctor recommended that I try an Atkins approach to losing weight. That meshed perfectly with my lifestyle, as well as with my underlying physical condition. And then there was a third miracle: I clicked on a link and joined an online dieting site, where I found support and coaching that worked for me.

Three miracles: a shift in perspective, the awareness that I could exert some control over my health via what I ate, and compassionate support around dieting, which included a diet plan that fit *me*. Without those things coming along right then in my life, I don't think I would be talking with you here today. I don't think I'd be helping women understand what's going on in their bodies and helping them survive and thrive through menopause. I wouldn't be planning my next adventure or getting ready to run my next half-marathon. I probably wouldn't be happily married, and I'm pretty sure I wouldn't be enjoying my body.

I also wouldn't be sure that this kind of transformation can happen for you, too. And I'm certain of that.

## THE REST OF THE STORY

It took me four years to achieve all the goals I set during that time when I decided not to check out, not to die. Some of them I achieved right away. Others took longer. In those four years, I started running (and ran numerous 5k and half-marathon races), learned to whitewater kayak and mountain bike, went skydiving and scuba diving, and fell in love. I lost 80 pounds. Since then, I've continued to make new goals and achieve them.

During and after those four years, I still had occasional menopausal symptoms, but they were mostly mild. I think that as you go through this book, you'll understand why my symptoms didn't stick around long enough to bother me (after all, I was my first client!). For example, at one point I got an intense case of the "itchies" and my bottle of lotion was my best friend. At the time, I also had a complete inability to concentrate on or care about the work I did in my job every day. Top that off with the reappearance of restless leg syndrome — a symptom I'd had earlier that had disappeared when I became a runner. I knew something was wrong. Again. I wasn't in the same place, physically, emotionally, or mentally, that I'd been in four years earlier, so I knew I needed to look around for different solutions.

I found myself increasingly drawn to helping the women in my dieting support group who were at the beginning of their menopausal journeys. I loved encouraging them and helping them figure out exercise and dietary plans. I loved that my running exploits were inspiring. I also loved going to the gym and helping the women there. I knew it was time to make a complete break from my corporate life. And so, I wound up studying personal training and running coaching, quitting my job, and starting to train women in the gym and "on the road" as runners.

That wasn't enough. I found that my favorite clients — women in their forties and fifties — were facing the same nutritional and lifestyle challenges I'd been faced with. The more research I did to help them create health in their lives, the more I felt that menopause and the hormonal changes that were happening in our bodies were at the root of almost every issue that women face in midlife. So I created Menopause Mastery Coaching.

## WHAT IS MENOPAUSE MASTERY COACHING?

I started doing what I do because *nobody* seemed to know anything about what's happening to them and nobody wanted to talk about it.

When I talk to women in their early forties, many of them don't even want to say the word "menopause," because that's about "old" people. And *they* obviously aren't old, because their periods are still perfectly regular. Menopause is years away. They often don't want to hear that they could experience a lot of symptoms later if they don't take better care of themselves now. They certainly don't want to figure out how to prepare for menopause by caring for themselves. They've got too much else to do right now!

When I talk with women in their mid-to-late forties, they're often aware that menopause is out there. For some, their doctor has told them, "You're not there yet." They spend a lot of time at their doctor's, though, because they're having all sorts of symptoms — from sore joints to heart palpitations. Nothing really appears on the tests that's conclusive, though, so instead of getting help with their hormonal issues, they're getting antidepressants.

Women in their early fifties tend to know more about perimenopause. They know or suspect that they're in it. But they still ask, "Is this perimenopause?" on a regular basis, because they're not really sure what perimenopause is or what the symptoms are. They're not sure where this path is heading and they don't feel any control over what's happening to their bodies, in their minds, and in their hearts. They don't understand how their hormones interact, how they're changing, and how they can manage those changes. They also don't understand how to bolster their overall experience.

Women in their mid-fifties may be hoping that *finally*, now that their periods have stopped, they'll get some relief. They end up in shock when, after their periods have stopped for over a year, some symptoms continue and new ones appear. They've been counting on that magic one-year marker to make everything better. They've been looking forward to being the person they used to be. But that doesn't always happen.

I also talk with women who are beyond menopause. Their reaction to what I do is usually something like, "Wow, I wish you'd been around when I was going through 'The Change!' I really could've used someone to talk to. Someone who actually *knew* what was happening. Someone who knew strategies that would have kept me from struggling so much."

What are the common threads among all these women, across all the phases of the menopause cycle? Women need information about what's happening during menopause, about why their bodies are behaving the way they are. Women need help to know how to support their bodies, both to manage the hormonal changes so they feel better and to continue to repair and renew, so they age appropriately. Above all, women want the chance to be their best self.

When we understand and embrace the changes that happen as a result of menopause, we can become the best versions of ourselves. Again.

# CHAPTER 2

# WHAT'S GOING ON IN YOUR BODY

I've got to warn you. There lies inside me, buried not too deep, a science geek. In fact, my friends tell me (sometimes rather pointedly), it's not buried at all! Some of the science stuff about menopause is really important for you to know, so my inner science geek is going to come out now and then. I'll try to give you fair warning and keep it to a minimum, but this science stuff is what helps you to understand why you're not going crazy, you're not going to die, and there is a plan here.

For a lot of you, the science may make your eyes glaze over long before my geek has played enough, but I've written what I think is the minimum you should know. Most of the geek is in this chapter and the next, but there are also a few bits and pieces scattered throughout the rest of the book.

In case you'd like more information, there are lots of additional details in the articles on my website, in a special section called *The Science Geek Speaks*. I add new stuff there all the time, so if you want to feed your inner science geek, check it out (www.menopause.guru/misg). There's even an *Ask the Science Geek* page, so you can ask a question and give me a chance to spend the morning doing my favorite thing — researching!

## THE DIFFERENCE BETWEEN
## BOYS AND GIRLS

So, let's start with the basics. How are men and women different?

There's the obvious outside stuff and there's not-so-obvious inside stuff and then there's the just-plain-annoying stuff (like how guys don't like to ask for directions and think you'd like a new vacuum cleaner for your birthday; and how gals get to be the ones with periods, pregnancy, and menopause). In biology class, they told us our differences are due to DNA: girls have double X chromosomes and boys have XY chromosomes, and that little half chromosome of difference is what does it all.

Well, not quite. It's true that boys having that Y chromosome makes a difference, but it's how our differences play out that creates all the uproar in your heart, mind, body, and spirit.

You see, men and women have different chemical environments because of the hormones put out by our endocrine systems. Men are dominated by testosterone and the other male, or *androgen*, hormones; women are dominated by the hormones estrogen and progesterone. Because the human body is designed to work fairly efficiently, all kinds of processes and even behaviors are tied to these hormones. Our differences are not only tied to our DNA, which remains the same throughout our lives, but also to lots of shifts as our inner hormonal environment changes, for throughout our lives.

## THE MIND AND THE BRAIN

Before we get too deep into hormones, let's take a moment and differentiate between the *mind* and the *brain*.

Your brain is that mass of cells inside your skull that monitors and controls *almost everything* that's happening in your body. Yes, it's the part that does your sensing, thinking, and feeling. And it controls all your movements. But it's also the part that's responsible for all the things you *don't* think about — your heart beating, digesting your food, and all those reproductive functions, like ovulating and menstruating.

Your brain communicates with the rest of you through three means: the *voluntary nervous system*, which controls things like movement and speech; the *autonomic nervous system*, which does all the housekeeping chores of keeping you running; and the *hormonal system*, which regulates and triggers a bunch of processes. All of these systems are built for two-way communication, and it's becoming clearer with recent research that the whole body is involved in intelligent communication with the brain.

The mind is harder to pin down. It's the part of you that does all the thinking and feeling; that interprets and constructs reality based on sensory and internal input; that remembers, decides, and acts. It's the part of you that's self-aware. There's also a level of responsibility the mind handles that you're likely not aware of, because those processes are usually happening subconsciously, though most can be brought into awareness by concentrating. Your mind often reacts to situations with an emotional response.

Your mind — the part of you that is aware and that decides to act — uses the same three communication avenues the brain uses. Primarily, the mind uses the voluntary pieces of the nervous system, but the mind can also influence and be influenced by the hormonal system and the autonomic nervous system.

Does that sound far-fetched? Here's a quick experiment. Think about something that scares you (for me, that's a snake, any snake). If you need to, look at a picture of the scary thing and let yourself get agitated by it. Feel your heart rate going up, your breaths getting shallower. Now close your eyes and think calming thoughts. Dispel the scary image and think instead about breathing slowly and deeply. Notice that your heart rate slows. You've just used your mind to affect your physical body.

This exercise is going to show up again later on in the book, so it's a great thing to try right now, to get a physical sense of how your mind can cause stress or calm stress, which it just did. There's lots more about this subject posted on my website, written by my Inner Science Geek. (www.menopause.guru/misg/category/mindbody).

## YOUR MENSTRUAL CYCLE

Unlike men, who manufacture sperm throughout their lives, women are born with all the reproductive material (eggs, or, more scientifically, *ova*) they're ever going to have. It's a huge number of eggs, but there's a high attrition rate, and only about 400 to 500 ova ever mature to the point that they could be fertilized (i.e., make a baby).

From the time we females hit puberty, our bodies think their primary job is to reproduce, so a lot of energy goes into that monthly cycle. The menstrual cycle consists of shedding the old uterine lining (menstruating), maturing the eggs (this takes place inside *follicles* in the ovaries), preparing the uterus with a new lining, releasing a single mature egg (ovulation), and, finally, colliding with a sperm cell (aka, fertilization) that causes a pregnancy, or, if the egg wasn't fertilized, shedding the uterine lining. This cycle takes about 28 days.

The two primary female hormones — progesterone and estrogen — are tied to the menstruation cycle. Progesterone is released when the egg is released, and estrogen is released as a result of the building and shedding of the uterine lining.

## THE STAGES OF MENOPAUSE

**Early Perimenopause.** Sometime in our late thirties or early forties, for most of us, *anovulatory cycles* (meaning menstrual cycles that don't include ovulation) start to happen. The egg that matures is not viable and fails to actually ovulate. In these cases, the follicle simply atrophies and dies without releasing progesterone. Even though no progesterone (or only minimal amounts) is released for that cycle, the uterine lining is still built and shed. Many women don't even notice they didn't ovulate. However, estrogen continues to be delivered, as usual, and you have your period. But the delicate balance between progesterone and estrogen has been upset. This is a state known as *estrogen dominance* and it causes its own set of effects (or symptoms) in your body. Many of these effects are similar to PMS (your body is in this state of estrogen dominance a couple of days each month during your regular cycle, anyway), but during perimenopause the effects of estrogen dominance may be more pronounced or continuous.

Early perimenopause may last for years, as you continue to have mostly normal periods, with occasional anovulatory cycles. This can be extremely annoying, because your doctor (especially your primary care or general practitioner) may not recognize your symptoms as perimenopause and the hormone tests may not show anything, especially if you aren't symptomatic when you see your doctor and the blood work is done.

Unfortunately, the shifting hormone balances of perimenopause can cause some annoying effects, many of which are mood-affecting. Depression, anxiety, and the inability to cope with the increased stress can make you feel like you're going crazy, and to have your doctor confirm that possibility (because neither you nor your doctor recognize the signs of perimenopause) is heart-wrenching.

**Late Perimenopause.** By this point, anovulatory cycles are the norm and your periods are probably *wonky* — that's a very official technical term — meaning you never know *what's* going to happen! (Don't wear white pants.) Not as much estrogen is produced during late perimenopause, especially during those "missed" periods. Progesterone is starting to bottom out. The effects of the hormonal shift are pretty well full-blown by now.

Other hormonal systems in the body — especially those involving the adrenal glands (cortisol and adrenal hormones), the pancreas (insulin), and the thyroid gland (thyroid hormones) — are also being affected by the lowered levels of estrogen and progesterone in your body. And yet that one part of the brain, the part that's controlled ovulation all along, still wants us to keep on having babies. (Bad, bad brain. No more 2 a.m. feedings, please!) The pituitary gland pumps out FSH (follicle stimulating hormone) at an even faster rate during late perimenopause, trying to get us to ovulate. It's that elevated FSH level that tells your doctor definitively that you're in perimenopause. (Well, duh, doc! Glad you finally see it my way!)

Now you know. Even if your doctor is *really* old school (old school says perimenopause refers to only that year when your periods have stopped, the year before the first anniversary of your last period), it will be obvious to him or her now that your body is telling you your reproductive system is shutting down.

Because your hormones are shifting far faster and more drastically than since puberty, you may feel great one moment and completely horrible the next. Mood shifts, hot flashes, anxiety, weird sensations — any of the symptoms related to rapid shifting in your body chemistry — become prevalent during this period.

You could easily be thrown off balance by the unpredictability of your cycles during this phase, especially if your menstrual cycle was highly regular before. Skipped periods, light periods, extremely heavy or long periods, and short or long cycles are all considered normal — and obnoxious — during late perimenopause.

To top it all off, you're still fertile, and you may be hit with the overwhelming desire to get pregnant. That wish happened to me (dang, I even named her — she was going to be Olivia) and it's happened to many of the women I've worked with. When your period doesn't show up, you may take that pregnancy test with half-hope and half-dread.

**Menopause.** Menopause is an event, an anniversary, a one-particular-day happening that I choose to celebrate with my clients. It's the first anniversary of the first day of your last period. That's the point at which you should be able to expect that you'll never have another period. Just a quick note, though. You shouldn't have another period, so if you do, let your doctor know. Usually it's nothing to be concerned about, but it should be checked.

Menopause is a marker that you've turned another page in your life's story. For many women, this is a celebration. It marks a time in their life when they get to concentrate on themselves, perhaps for the first time in their lives.

Menopause also means that your hormones are beginning to settle into a non-cyclic level that's your new normal for the rest of your life. At this point, most women begin to see a change in the symptoms they feel, and many of the symptoms they do experience are those more associated with aging, not hormonal changes.

You can also quit using birth control when you reach menopause, because, in all likelihood, you'll never ovulate again. (Yes, there's probably the unusual case out there where pregnancy happened after that year, but it's extremely rare.) For some of you, especially those whose ambitions for children went unfulfilled, this may be a melancholy realization.

**Postmenopause.** Postmenopause begins after that one-year marker of menopause and lasts for the rest of your life. It's a gradual transition from the ending of menstrual cycles to full adjustment to the hormonal levels that are left. It's also a period when all of you — your heart, mind, and spirit — begins to realize what's possible in life for you, and to consider what you want to do with the years and decades you have left.

During the first two years of postmenopause or so, your body begins to settle in, to adjust to its new levels of hormones. Your adrenal glands and your fat cells do most of the estrogen production for you now, producing at about ten percent of your premenopausal levels. Your ovaries still do some hormone production as well, and that seems to provide some residual modulating effects. (Research in this area is sorely lacking, but it's clear that having ovaries into postmenopause is better for you than not having them, unless there's a specific medical reason to have them removed).

Your progesterone levels are very low now, and most of what's there is made in the adrenal glands, not the ovaries.

In general, the symptoms of estrogen dominance go away and symptoms may occur that have to do with low levels of female hormones. While the symptoms of low estrogen and low progesterone are often considered "signs of aging," they can feel new and odd for women going through this phase. Symptoms can include: osteoporosis; dry and aging skin; weight gain (especially around the middle); crawling, itching skin; and vaginal changes (especially dryness and atrophy). Unfortunately, some of your old friends from perimenopause may hang around, too, especially hot flashes.

A lot of women who are struggling with perimenopause give the day marking their menopause — the day they've gone 365 days without a period — an almost mystical meaning. They believe that on day one of postmenopause they'll be transported into a magic, never-ever-again land where all their symptoms are gone and everything is wonderful.

The reality is, there is no magic land. You adjust, slowly or quickly, to the body you have now. That body is something to be cherished and nourished, because it can still do marvelous and amazing things if you support it.

Here's a small example. Recently, I joined a group of close to 50 women to kayak the Nantahala River, a Class II-III whitewater river in North Carolina. The women ranged in age from 19 to over 70. At the end of the day, I talked with one woman in her seventies who had rowed an oar boat down instead of taking her kayak. I asked her why. Her reply? "I need the practice. We leave for the Grand Canyon in two weeks, and I'm taking the oar boat down." WOW! I was speechless! (Piloting an oar boat through the Grand Canyon isn't easy at *any* age!) And I have a new role model.

* * *

That's the *how* regarding your body's changes through the stages of menopause — how the hormones are different in your body from one stage to the next. Hopefully, I've given you some insight into what's already happened in your body and what might happen next.

Take a deep breath and relax. In the next chapter, I'm going to continue with the science stuff and tell you what else estrogen and progesterone do, besides controlling menstrual cycles and nurturing babies.

Together, this chapter and the next one provide the background for the rest of the book, in which we'll take a look at what's happening in each of those four big areas of your life — body, heart (emotions), mind (and brain), and spirit — and what you can do to feel better, look better, and be healthier in each of those areas.

# CHAPTER 3

# EVERYTHING'S CONNECTED

Now that we've talked about what happens during your menstrual cycle, let's look at what goes on in your hormonal system as a result.

## HORMONES, AND NEUROTRANSMITTERS, AND GLANDS, OH MY!

We often hear things like, "Oh, look at all those women fanning themselves. Are *all* of them having hot flashes? Hormones!" or, "Those out-of-control teenagers — raging hormones!" If you thought about those kinds of statements, you'd think all hormones were "sex hormones." But there are about 50 *known* hormones in the human body (I say "known" because we seem to still be discovering them!).

What are hormones and what do they do? Hormones are "regulatory substances produced in an organism and transported in tissue fluids such as blood to stimulate specific cells or tissues into action" (definition from the *New Oxford American Dictionary*). The *precursors* of all those hormones, what the body uses to make its hormones, are taken in in the same way the body absorbs the vast majority of its raw materials (except air) for the business of life, through the food we eat. Organs with the primary job of producing hormones are usually called *glands*. But glands aren't the only things that produce hormones; other organs, such as the uterus, ovaries, liver and even the brain, also produce hormones.

Hormones don't stay where they were made. They travel throughout your body, regulating processes at all levels and often having more than one job. Hormones are one of the main ways that your body communicates with itself, and levels of specific hormones can change in an instant. When hormones affect brain activity, they're often known as *neurotransmitters* and can change how you think, feel, and react.

## WHICH HORMONES ARE INVOLVED IN MENOPAUSE?

It's quite possible that there are many interactions that haven't yet been discovered between female sex hormones and other hormones. When we talk about symptoms, you'll see that there are some interactions that scientists don't understand. Neither do we! But the interactions below are the ones that have been found to be directly involved with and affected by menopausal shifts.

**Progesterone and Estrogen.** The primary source for both of these "female" hormones during our reproductive years are the ovaries and the ovulation process. Both progesterone and estrogen are by-products of the ovulation cycle. As more cycles become anovulatory (see Chapter Two), our ovaries produce first less progesterone and then less estrogen. Apparently, after menopause, no progesterone is produced in the ovaries, but a small amount of estrogen still continues to be produced.

Progesterone and estrogen are also both produced in our adrenal glands; this is true for both men and women. After menopause, residual amounts continue to be produced in the adrenals. Belly fat is another source of estrogen in both men and women. After menopause, having a small amount of belly fat — increasing your ideal weight by about ten pounds — actually makes sense for hormone production, and allows you to relax a bit about weight gain!

**Follicle Stimulating Hormone (FSH) and Luteinizing Hormone (LH).** These hormones are produced in the pituitary gland (in the brain) and begin increasing as anovulatory cycles become more common. By late perimenopause, both of these hormones stabilize at a level about two times their premenopausal maximum. Very little research seems to have been done on the physical or other (mental, emotional, etc.) effects of these hormones, so I won't speculate on anything they might do, other than one thing, the reason I include them in this list: Most doctors rely on the levels of FSH in the bloodstream to "diagnose" perimenopause. The problem with relying on this test is that if you are in an ovulatory cycle when the blood is drawn and most of your cycles are "normal," your levels may not register as perimenopausal. Does this mean perimenopause hasn't started for you? No. It just means the tests aren't very accurate.

If your doctor uses hormonal testing as only one of the tools in her or his arsenal to figure out where you are on your journey, keep him or her! This doctor is a gem beyond price! I've helped dozens of women find what works for them to ease their symptoms, despite their doctors telling them they weren't in perimenopause. This is because I rely on reported symptoms to figure out what's going on hormonally, and then work with women to help them make natural changes like improving nutrition, increasing movement, and reducing stress in order to promote health.

Oh, and by the way, there *are* many good doctors out there who understand this stuff. Some of them are gynecologists or family practitioners. But, if you're not getting what you need from them, your best bet in your area may be a gynecologist who specializes in menopause or a functional or integrative medicine specialist, a naturopath, or other alternative medicine practitioner. Ask your friends and look at references to find your best choice in your area.

**Cortisol.** Cortisol is the stress hormone that has gotten so much press, especially for its role in creating belly fat. It is made in the adrenal glands, along with the other adrenal hormones (epinephrine and norepinephrine), androgens (male hormones that women also have), and female hormones. From what's been published about cortisol, you may be wanting to totally eliminate it from your body. But cortisol is crucial. It has two primary jobs. The first is to keep you moving through the days as it works with your *circadian rhythms* (the natural wake/sleep cycle) to provide more stimulation during the day and less at night. Your adrenal glands will always produce at least the amount of cortisol needed to support that wake/sleep cycle before it produces anything else.

The second function of cortisol is to respond to medium-to-long-term stress by preparing your body to "dig in" for a long fight. Immediate responses to danger are handled by epinephrine, but if the stress is longer than momentary, cortisol takes over. When stress levels stay high over the long term, the adrenal glands may not be able to produce as much cortisol as your body thinks you need. If you continue to need it, your adrenals may become so over-worked they no longer function sufficiently. This is a state known as *adrenal fatigue* (and it's still controversial among doctors. Some don't want to recognize it as a *real* disease or syndrome.).

We weren't designed to deal with never-ending amounts of stress. The way our bodies are designed, stress should disappear in fairly short order. The body interprets long-term elevated cortisol levels as "famine" — the most common type of long-term stress our bodies used to go through, from an evolutionary perspective. Whenever there's enough food, the body socks it away as fat, because you never know where your next meal is coming from. But if the body thinks it's in famine mode, and since we almost always have extra food around... well, you know what happens: weight gain.

Once the adrenals become incapable of producing enough cortisol to keep up with the demand of our over-stressed bodies, we're stuck with a new problem. The source of our "get up and go" has, as they say, "got up and went." And because the adrenals see producing cortisol as the most important of their duties, everything else that's supposed to be produced (progesterone, estrogen, the androgens, epinephrine) are all placed on hold. (I'll say more about the effects of this later).

**Insulin.** Insulin is produced in your pancreas and is what regulates blood sugar — the amount of sugar that is circulating in your body and available to cells for quick energy. The appropriate level of sugar is a fairly narrow range. Too little, and you become quickly fatigued, or even faint. Too much, and your cells begin to be poisoned by sugar.

Insulin works to get the sugar extracted from food through the digestive process, stored either in cells that need it, or as fat cells for later use. If there's not enough energy coming in, insulin directs fat cells to release energy into the bloodstream to provide the energy you need.

Your body wants to use what you consume for its current needs: sugars and fats for energy and proteins and fat for building and repairing tissue. Insulin directs this process. If your cells are rarely in need of replenishing, a condition known as *insulin resistance* occurs. This means that the default action for the stuff you eat is to store it as fat and to have too much sugar circulating in the bloodstream for too long, which eventually leads to Type 2 Diabetes.

Type 2 Diabetes is the inability of your body to properly process blood-borne sugar. Type 2 Diabetes can be extremely dangerous, but is highly correctable through diet and exercise.

**Thyroid Hormones.** The thyroid gland, which is located at the base of your throat, produces the thyroid hormones T3, and T4. Thyroid stimulating hormone (TSH), which regulates the production of thyroid hormones, is produced in the pituitary gland. T3, the active version of the thyroid hormone, is responsible for regulating your metabolism. It controls how fast you burn sugar, fat, or protein for energy, how you make proteins, and how other hormones function. In many ways, the thyroid gland is the master gland for how your body runs. T4, the inactive version of the thyroid hormone, is converted to T3 "on the fly." TSH is the hormone that tells your thyroid you need more T3 and T4.

Unfortunately, a number of things can go wrong in this process. The thyroid can be damaged and not produce enough hormones. There can be problems with converting T4 to T3. There can be problems with cells being able to process T3, creating a *thyroid resistant* condition throughout your body.

And, prior to there being actual thyroid damage, thyroid functioning can just get sluggish. One of the most common causes of that is yo-yo dieting, which convinces the body that there's never a constant food supply, so it had better slow down on burning calories.

**Androgens.** Androgens are the so-called *male hormones*. Just as men have estrogen and progesterone (but at much lower levels than we do), we have male hormones at lower levels than men. Our supply of androgens is made primarily in our adrenal glands. There are several different androgens. Testosterone is the best known and, in women, accounts for some of our sex drive, as well as mood regulation (avoiding depression), keeping energy levels sustainable, brain and bone health, building and maintaining muscle, and other important bodily processes.

In addition to testosterone, there are also DHEA (Dehydroepiandrosterone), DHT (dihydrotestosterone), and androsterone. Because we are women, there's a fairly narrow "right" range of these male hormones for us. Too little and we become dragged out, tired, and a bit lackluster. Too much (or too much in relation to our estrogen and progesterone levels), and we get "fun" symptoms such as acne, male-pattern baldness, and hair growth in other unwanted places (the dreaded chin hairs and moustache).

**Neurotransmitters.** Neurotransmitters help your brain operate correctly by promoting various processes, such as sleep, and by regulating your moods. Some of the neurotransmitters affected by menopause include:

- **Melatonin.** This is the sleep neurotransmitter. When it's working right, it increases with the onset of darkness and lessens towards morning, setting up a good sleep cycle. It works in conjunction with cortisol to regulate your sleep-wake cycles.

- **Serotonin.** One of the "feel-good" hormones, serotonin helps regulate appetite, sleep, and mood. Low serotonin is one of the common causes of depression.

- **Dopamine.** This neurotransmitter operates as a reward for behavior perceived as positive by the brain. Addictions are often the result of increased dopamine rewarding the use of a substance.

- **Oxytocin.** This is the love (or bonding) hormone. It is released upon cuddling or bonding (especially during mother/infant bonding or during sex) and is a powerful "feel-good" hormone.

- **Norepinephrine.** Produced in the adrenals, this is the excitement hormone that makes the things just this side of fearful seem fun. For some of us, it's a merry-go-round or a Ferris wheel that triggers production of this hormone; for others, it's a roller coaster or a bungee jump.

## CONNECTIONS AND COMPLICATIONS

Why are all of these hormones and chemicals so affected by changes in your menstrual cycle? And why should you care about them and what they do?

Well, it turns out that hormones are highly interactive, and how one acts on your body is often dependent on the levels of other hormones. What this means is that a change in the level of one hormone can easily affect every cell, every organ, and every system in your body. And that seems to be especially true of the way estrogen works.

These complex hormonal interactions are a large part of what creates the changes and side effects (aka, symptoms) of menopause. During the menopausal journey, our hormones are shifting (especially progesterone and estrogen) to a new normal. By the time you reach menopause, progesterone and estrogen will be at very low levels compared to the levels they were during your reproductive years.

On the way to that new state, there will be a number of fluctuations and temporary imbalances. I want to explore some of the major ones for two reasons. The first is that your symptoms are caused by what's not in balance, either in the relationships between hormones or in terms of optimum levels of hormones. By looking at what's going on in your life, you can make an educated guess as to what's happening in your body and with your hormones.

And that leads us to the all-important second reason. If you know what's out of balance, you can take steps to bring it back into balance. Many of the methods I help my clients use to bring themselves into balance — so that they're feeling great, losing weight, and looking terrific! — are found in the rest of this book.

Menopausal symptoms relating to different hormonal imbalances can be found on my website (www.menopause. guru/symptoms). There's a lot of overlap between various imbalances, and new relationships between symptoms and imbalances are constantly discovered, so when I work with clients to figure out what's going on, we look at symptom patterns, along with menstrual patterns and their own intuition, to pick a place to start in correcting them.

So, what are these hormone imbalances and deficiencies? Let's take a look.

**Low Progesterone.** As I've said, beginning in early perimenopause, progesterone levels can decrease significantly and fluctuate depending on ovulation. Progesterone is one of the imbalances that is least affected by the types of lifestyle changes I generally recommend. If the symptoms of low progesterone are severe, there are bioidentical hormones available to help.

**Low Estrogen.** Estrogen starts to drop during perimenopause. For some women, it fluctuates wildly, while for others it drops fairly steadily until it reaches its new level. Estrogen levels can be optimized both during perimenopause and afterwards. However, there may be limits to how much you can optimize, and additional support through hormone replacement therapy (HRT) may be needed.

**Estrogen dominance.** Estrogen dominance occurs when progesterone has dropped and is low relative to estrogen (estrogen levels themselves can be low, normal, or high). Estrogen dominance tends to be a problem in perimenopause, but the symptoms often disappear after menopause, when estrogen settles at a low level. It is possible that symptoms of both low estrogen and estrogen dominance can be present at once, since estrogen dominance is the relationship of estrogen to progesterone.

**(Relatively) High Testosterone.** In general, unless a woman has high testosterone to begin with, this imbalance happens when testosterone levels remain the same and estrogen drops. Estrogen "opposes" testosterone, which means it balances out the effects of testosterone and keeps most women from experiencing complications from high testosterone before perimenopause. When estrogen drops, testosterone can cause the symptoms associated with high testosterone in women (such as acne, stray hairs, and thinning hair).

**Low Testosterone.** For some women, especially those under a lot of stress, menopause signals a lowering of the production of testosterone. This brings its own set of symptoms, including loss of muscle mass and bone, fatigue, and lowered sex drive.

**High Cortisol or Adrenal Fatigue.** Estrogen modulates your body's response to cortisol. It actually helps you cope with stress. The process of menopause, the changes the body goes through, the hormone and chemical fluctuations, the symptoms — all create their own stresses. Add those stresses to the stress of navigating modern life, having kids in college, managing aging parents, and all the rest, and cortisol can rise to extremely high levels.

If you don't do anything to control high cortisol levels (see Chapter Seven), your adrenals can get pushed to the point where they no longer function properly. This results in cortisol levels that are too low (aka, adrenal fatigue), along with lowered levels of estrogen, progesterone, androgens, epinephrine, and norepinephrine.

**High Insulin and/or Insulin Resistance.** Estrogen affects insulin, helping it to work better. After estrogen begins to drop, insulin doesn't work as well and you are more at risk for insulin resistance. The symptoms of insulin resistance often go unnoticed, but insulin resistance is the first step on the path to Type 2 Diabetes.

**Low Thyroid Function.** Estrogen is a factor here, too. Are you sensing a pattern? You should be! Estrogen is a huge factor in how almost all processes in your body work. Low estrogen can affect the thyroid receptors on cells, with the result that, even with good thyroid levels in your bloodstream, your metabolism doesn't work right.

The bad news doesn't end there. High cortisol can interrupt thyroid functioning. So can a lot of environmental factors. So can yo-yo dieting or very low-calorie dieting.

**Neurotransmitters.** And, finally, all those neurotransmitters? Yep, those, too. Fluctuations in estrogen and cortisol interfere with neurotransmitters as well. Melatonin doesn't work as well — so we sleep badly (and high cortisol interferes even more). Serotonin, dopamine, and oxytocin are all produced at lower levels and so don't work as well. Norepinephrine, which comes from the adrenals, is produced in smaller amounts when cortisol is in high demand, and so we feel "flat," unable to get excited about our lives.

## THE BAD NEWS

The bad news is that every cell in our bodies — in our brains, all our muscles, organs, and bones — is affected by the process of menopause. Because menopause takes years to complete, its symptoms can go on and on and keep changing as the imbalances shift.

I've given basic explanations above for why so many things are tied to the changes of menopause and why your experience can be so different from that of your sister, your best friend, or, certainly, your mother.

Doctors can be stymied by the complexity of menopause's symptoms and that same complexity is why hormone replacement therapy might not be the best choice for *your* set of symptoms.

## THE GOOD NEWS

If telling you all of that was just a long-winded way of breaking bad news to you — of telling you that you're going to feel miserable for the rest of your life — I promise I wouldn't be writing this book. I'd be sitting in a corner somewhere, feeling miserable and anticipating feeling that way forever. But I'm not.

I *do* have good news for you! Even though these imbalances can seem hopelessly complex and ever-present, there are things that can work to help you feel better, to help you balance your hormones and get healthier (and happier) than you may have been for a long time.

There is a myriad of ways of achieving a new, healthy you. For most women, those ways don't need to involve pharmaceuticals, surgery, or exotic herbs. The side-effects of those solutions can sometimes be as devastating as the symptoms you are trying to treat. Plus, they often don't address the underlying causes: the hormonal imbalances.

There are times when drugs, surgery, or herbs are extremely helpful. For some women, there are times when the symptoms get so overwhelming that they endanger their health, their primary relationships or their jobs. Then, it can be beneficial to work with a physician who understands the need to recapture hormonal balance, together with making the lifestyle changes that support on-going wellness.

In the rest of this book, I'm going to show you how I work with women to help them change the way they feel, to recapture their zest and joy for life, and to begin seeing the beautiful path they want to follow for this next phase of their life.

I'll suggest new ways of looking at the things you're feeling, to see if you can use your symptoms to improve your worldview. We'll look at the big picture — your heart, your mind, your physical being, and your spiritual life — and explore how menopause opens up new aspects of each of these. You can take the child you were, the young woman you became, and the mature woman you are becoming and put them all together into a sensational new you.

I'll provide you with the same techniques I teach my clients, so you can make changes in your lifestyle to support the woman you are and the woman you're becoming. I'll tell you about the nutrition, movement, and stress management techniques my clients have used to lose weight, become more fit, and become calmer, happier, and more fulfilled than ever before.

But, we all know change can be hard and menopause can create so much havoc in our lives. When we're left to our own devices, making even *more* changes may be too hard. The support we get in our journey often makes the difference! So I'll also show you how to get the support you need to make it all happen.

# THE CAVEATS

Symptoms of perimenopause and postmenopause vary widely among women. Some women sail through, and really don't even notice until their periods have been missing for a few months. Others have symptoms of such intensity that they cannot function without medical intervention. There seems to be no way to predict where you're going to be on that spectrum.

Only you and your medical professional can decide what's right for you. For some women, that means using lifestyle and mindset changes to bolster their health and well-being. For others, that means medical intervention, either through hormone replacement therapy or other drugs which have been shown to provide relief for specific symptoms or sets of symptoms. For some women, surgery is the best course of treatment.

If you are unable to function in your daily life or your symptoms are threatening your primary relationships, I urge you to take action to make some changes. Whether it's natural or medical treatments, please get the help you need to be happier and healthier. Because that's what it's all about.

This book is written for women who choose to follow, as much as possible, a path through menopause that relies primarily on lifestyle and mindset changes. Even there, I encourage my clients to have a close, personal relationship with a medical practitioner who can help them find the right support should they need it. Sometimes, that's for a short period of time; other times, the support may be longer-term, or even permanent.

Each woman is different, and you must travel the path that's right for you. Whatever path you choose, know that I'm cheering for you!

# CHAPTER 4

# HOW HORMONAL CHANGES AFFECT YOU

Perimenopause can seem to start out of nowhere. We're going along, living our lives, knowing what to expect each month with our menstrual cycles — whether that's good, bad, or really ugly. Then, things change. We never know from day to day how we'll feel in our bodies or how we'll feel emotionally. The way we think changes. So much is affected by the changes of menopause.

Every day, I talk with women who are trying to figure out what's happening to them, when it's going to be over, and what the end result is going to be. Are they going to be able to feel happy and be healthy? Are they ever going to feel like themselves again?

In this chapter, I'll tell you more about what all those changes I introduced in the previous two chapters actually do to your body, to your emotions, and to your mind. About how those changes make you feel. And then we'll get busy with what can help you feel better — and maybe even beyond better.

# THE "NORMAL" PATH THROUGH MENOPAUSE

There is no normal. Every woman's path is going to be a little different. There are so many factors involved that it's almost impossible to predict what's going to happen when.

To further complicate matters, there are all those other hormones besides the primary two — progesterone and estrogen — that affect the stages of menopause. Add the possibility of thyroid, insulin, cortisol, and testosterone imbalances to the changes in estrogen and progesterone and you get dozens of symptoms in millions of combinations. No one has an exact list of all the symptoms associated with the process of menopause, but the most common lists catalog 33, 34, 66, or 117 symptoms.

While even the smallest of those lists is tremendously depressing, it's pretty rare for one woman to have all of those symptoms at once, or even in her lifetime. Some women will report no symptoms except the cessation of their periods. Others will claim they're going through all the symptoms at once. Most women experience several symptoms at any one time, and then those disappear to be replaced by new ones.

The thing that's most true is that almost every odd and annoying symptom you feel in your body during this time is related to or intensified by the changing hormones we've talked about. If you don't consider menopause as the source of most of your symptoms, you may spend a lot of time anxious about a medical issue that doesn't really exist. I call this the *Peruvian Shepherd Boy Disease Syndrome*. Here's how it works: You feel lousy. Maybe you're itching. It feels like ants crawling on your skin. You run to the computer, flip it on and google your symptoms. There it is! What you're experiencing is the first symptom of a rare disease contracted by shepherds living above 7000 feet in the Andes. The crawling ants feeling will be followed by flushing (and now you have a hot flash). Suddenly you're convinced that even though you live in Nebraska and you've never met a Peruvian shepherd, you've contracted this disease, from which you'll die a horrible death. In three weeks.

But if, instead, you'd googled, say, "itching crawling skin menopause," you could have found information about *formication*, the feeling of ants crawling on (or under) your skin, a symptom of menopause associated with low estrogen. Oh, whew! Relax. The condition is obnoxious, but not fatal.

I don't want to say that there's never a symptom that's not related to menopause. It's important to keep in touch with your doctors and explore anything that you feel might be serious, but if you start with the assumption that it's a symptom of perimenopause or menopause, you get to relax until your doctor tells you something really is wrong.

## A CAVEAT ABOUT SYMPTOMS

I'm not going to list every symptom or possible symptom as I tell you about what you can do to ease your own symptoms. When I first started thinking about this book and what and how to tell you about all the possible symptoms, I wanted to describe them and tell you when they happened and what they feel like and what you could do about them. But then I realized that I could spend 200 pages describing the common and not-so-common symptoms that *might* affect you.

And you'd be scared. You'd be checking your skin and freaking out over every stray hair in your hairbrush. If you experienced *tinnitus*, a ringing in your ears that's a common occurrence in perimenopause, you'd be terrified that maybe you had a brain tumor. You might overanalyze every belch, every tummy rumble, and every difference in your period, asking yourself, "Is this a symptom? How long is it going to bother me?"

Then again, you might have none of the 117-plus symptoms. And I would have contributed to you wasting your time and energy worrying about things that probably won't happen and aren't really that bad anyway.

So I decided to take a different tack in this book and not get specific about a big list of possible symptoms. Even if you're annoyed by multiple symptoms, most of them aren't going to be health-threatening, much less life-threatening.

I'm not writing this book to scare you! If you want explanations of each and every symptom associated with the stages of menopause, there are resources out there. You can, for example, go to my website to see a list of symptoms and the hormonal imbalances they're associated with (www.menopause.guru/symptoms).

What I would like to give you here, instead, is a more general overview of how the hormonal changes you're going through may be affecting you. I won't tell you that your symptoms are "all in your head" or "not as bad as you're making them out to be," because some of them can be downright debilitating. Even the ones that *are* "all in your head" — like depression, anxiety, and mood swings — have a physiological basis in your hormonal imbalances.

In the following chapters, I'll tell you about simple, practical changes you can make to "change the change" — to make it possible for you to stop seeing menopause as a curse or an illness.

## BODIES INHABITED BY ALIENS

Often, the first symptoms of perimenopause we notice are the physical ones. There can be a lot of them. They may appear and disappear, and it can feel like there's no rhyme or reason to the way your body feels from one day to the next. Your every cell is affected by perimenopause, so all kinds of bizarre symptoms can appear.

What this reminds me of is the movie *Alien*. I admit that I've never seen the movie (I'm not a horror movie kinda person), but if you were alive in 1979 when the movie came out, it was hard to miss the concept: Human space travelers encounter an alien life form that uses the astronauts' bodies to incubate its young. Something else — an alien life form — took charge of the inhabited body.

Yep, that's the way perimenopause can feel. Whether you loved your body or not before these changes began, you were probably comfortable enough with it. You knew what to expect. You had an idea of when your period was coming. You knew which days of your menstrual cycle were most likely to make you feel lousy and which days made you feel great. You knew there'd be that day when your "fat jeans" would come out, but you also knew you'd be back to normal (whether you were satisfied with your "normal" or not) in a day or three. You knew what to do if you had an event coming up where you wanted to look your best, and you could maybe drop a few pounds using your favorite diet. The condition of your hair and skin was predictable. You had a routine.

*And then.*

And then your body started changing without warning (or at least without anything you recognized as a warning!). The predictability — your routine — was gone.

Some of the changes of perimenopause you might notice early on are those caused by low progesterone and/or estrogen dominance. These changes can include menstrual irregularities, which, for you, may even look like more regular periods. These symptoms can also feel a lot like PMS, which maybe you've never had, but which now accompanies every period. Or maybe you've always had PMS, but now it's even worse.

Later in perimenopause and in postmenopause, you may experience symptoms associated with low estrogen. Estrogen is our "juicy" hormone — the one that seems to keep our bodies lubricated in lots of different ways. Many of the symptoms of low estrogen feel like "drying out": dry skin and nails and hair. Osteoporosis. Vaginal drying.

The symptoms of high cortisol include feelings of being stressed out. Low cortisol symptoms are similar to those of low thyroid: feeling dragged out and exhausted. Insulin resistance causes few noticeable symptoms, but you may notice increased belly fat, weight loss difficulties, and cravings.

Symptoms of other hormone imbalances can occur at almost any time, because changes in estrogen and progesterone levels can create other imbalances at any time. Other hormones (sometimes called *associated hormones*) can be out of balance for reasons having nothing to do with menopause, too.

Now let's take a look at how these hormonal changes affect your emotional life — your heart. And then we'll look at their effects on your mind and brain.

## HEARTS HIJACKED BY HORMONES

I call the emotional changes of menopause "hijacked by hormones," because that's what it feels like to me. The emotions I'm feeling at any one time don't seem to make any sense. Something other than me is in control of how I *feel* about things.

During perimenopause, your reactions to life's emotional situations may seem bigger, over the top, and much more volatile. One minute you're laughing and goofing off, being silly and happy. The next, you're in a rage, or weeping uncontrollably.

We're often told that "our thoughts create our emotions." Here's an example of how that works: Maybe, when you were a little girl, you liked to play outside, because that's where you could connect with your friends, but when it rained you had to play at home, and your mom wouldn't let your friends come over. So, rainy days were boring, and all you did was mope around until they were over. You didn't like it when it rained. Now, as an adult, when it rains, you don't feel like doing anything and you get mopey and you feel lonely.

But maybe your husband was raised differently. Maybe, in his household, his mom would get really excited when it rained. She'd let him put on a bathing suit and she and his siblings and friends would play outside in the rain and make mudpies, and then they'd all go back inside and bake cookies together. Now when it rains, your husband acts like that little kid again — happy and ready to play and wanting to connect.

Even if association memories like those don't come to the surface consciously enough to describe or to see the origins of, they're there. When you wake up and it's raining you might say to yourself, "Oh, damn. Another rainy day. I won't get anything done today. It's just miserable out and I feel just miserable." Meanwhile, there's your husband, bouncing out of bed, thinking, "*Rain!* Boy, what a great day today is going to be."

You and your husband have the same stimulus: a rainy day. But you have different thoughts about it that arise from different memories. The final result? You experience low energy (and maybe feel a bit resentful) and he dances through his day (and wonders what's wrong with you).

Now, take that same rainy day and throw in some hormonal changes. Instead of having low energy now, your reaction to the rain blooms into full-scale depression. Your husband's goofy attempts to cheer you up, which might have solicited a smile in the past, are now just irritating. The higher level of cortisol surging through your body triggers a rage reaction, and you yell at him, telling him to "Go away and just leave me alone!"

What's the cause of your reaction? You? Or the hormones? It's actually a bit of both: you reacting to a situation (the rainy day) that you don't like, and your hormones taking over and deepening that reaction. Your husband does what he always does, tries to tease you out of it. Maybe another thought down there, so deep down you may not be aware of thinking it, jumps into the fray. Maybe it's the thought, "I wish he'd just let me feel what I want to feel" or "That's such a corny joke, and he's told it a zillion times before." This causes stress, the cortisol takes over in reaction to your stress, and you veer out of control.

Emotionally, you're shifting all over the place. Much of that happens because your brain chemistry has changed.

## MINDS MISSING IN ACTION

Here's another menopause cliché: We wander from room to room, doing part of a chore here, stopping to do something else there, then another thing over there. But we never seem to circle back and finish anything. UGH!

Why does that happen? What's causing it?

As women going through our reproductive years, our biology, our hormones, tended to make us natural caretakers. Even those of us who didn't become mothers. The nature of caregiving is that it's tough to schedule it. You start helping with one thing here, then jump over there to take care of a sudden need, then fix some other situation that needs a tweak, then handle an emergency. Estrogen helps our brains do that *serial-tasking* thing. (Many people think of it as multi-tasking, but it's really cyclical serial-tasking.) It helps us keep track of where we were in each chore and keeps us circling back to complete everything. (Don't worry if this never described you — but you were probably still better at this kind of serial-tasking than most of your male acquaintances.)

As estrogen retreats during perimenopause, we try to continue to serial-task (because it's a habit), but feel like we're failing miserably at it. We feel like we never get anything completed. We forget stuff and our organizing or list systems that used to work now seem ineffective at keeping us on track. On the other hand, now we may be better straight-line thinkers — more able to concentrate on single tasks without interruption, even if we have to practice this new type of thinking to get good at it.

In what other ways do our brains change as we enter the stages of menopause?

The brain's communication center runs on estrogen. Even before we were born, estrogen helped us developed stronger verbal skills than males. Estrogen helps us read faces and communicate, both non-verbally and verbally. And then, during perimenopause, we're suddenly stuck trying to find a word — that word we were just thinking of a minute ago. Or we forget the names of people we've known forever. It has us wondering if we're going crazy or developing Alzheimer's.

Estrogen also helps us care what others think about us and want to protect our relationships (sometimes at way too great a cost to ourselves), so that we have a safe haven in which to raise our children. Estrogen makes us want to connect with others and preserve those connections. When estrogen diminishes, we may stop being as interested in being the peacemaker and the social butterfly.

Our natural inclination as these changes occur is to not care as much about our social relationships. We may even shock ourselves with how little we care about others' opinions. We may hesitate to take on social obligations, even ones that brought us great joy before.

Last October, one of my clients, Nancy, began a session by complaining for almost five minutes, without pause, about how little she was looking forward to "the holidays." About 15 years before, she'd taken over the big family Christmas party. An event that had once delighted her now filled her with dread. I suggested that perhaps 15 years ago her mom had been more than willing to give up her duties for the same reason Nancy was dreading the big party this year: menopausal changes.

I helped Nancy plan the transition of the responsibility for the holiday party to her daughter, Denise, and I also suggested that Nancy let her daughter know *why* she was tired of being the "hostess with the mostest," so that Denise could plan her own transition in a decade or so.

In a similar vein, when I suggested to another client, Kathy, that she re-do her Myers-Briggs assessment as part of our work together, she remembered her previous Myers-Briggs type as indicating she was, in part, an extrovert. Her new assessment, she was surprised to discover, showed that she now fell squarely on the introvert side of the scale.

Even what feels like a basic aspect of your personality may change as your brain chemistry reacts to the hormonal changes of menopause.

## SPIRITS DAMPENED AND DISCOURAGED

I found myself discouraged and disheartened after my marriage fell apart. I wanted to be happy and to be looking forward to the rest of my life. I wanted to think that life could be awesome still. But, I didn't really believe it. And I certainly didn't feel it.

What I felt was that I was losing myself. I had lost my zest for life, my interest in the things I'd loved before, and even the way I felt about my family wasn't the same.

*I just wanted to be me again!*

It was more than my body, my mind, and my emotions — I felt I was losing the very core of who I was. And, in the years that have followed, I see so many of the women I interact with feeling exactly the same.

Even if you've made a powerful and exciting life for yourself, menopause can turn that on its head. Menopause means that we're coming to the end of one chapter and beginning a new one. It means leaving some things behind (especially childbearing), and finding a new way to be in the world.

It can be scary. Traditionally, menopause is the province of "old women," of crones and hags. We can feel like life is almost over and we get scared that we haven't accomplished all that we've wanted to do. We're still adding items to our bucket list, and there are so many things on there that we haven't had a chance to do, to be, and even to have. What we often don't see is that menopause has a message for us.

## THE MESSAGE OF MENOPAUSE: IT'S TIME FOR YOU!

There are tons of things going on with your body that seem odd now. If you're like me, you find yourself looking to doctors for advice more than you ever have before, but coming away with few answers to the issues bothering you. If you're lucky, you'll be "diagnosed" as perimenopausal. But you already knew that, right? When you think about it, you may realize that you didn't need a doctor to tell you that.

Your doctor may offer you drugs to make you feel better. He or she might recommend antidepressants or other mood altering drugs. In some cases, you and your doctor may feel you're really need them right now. But those drugs have all kinds of side effects, and they dampen the good feelings as well as the bad, so there's a tradeoff. Carefully consider if they are the right decision for you.

Or maybe your doctor recommends hormone replacement therapy (HRT). The problem is that HRT may not be effective for your specific symptoms. Most doctors will only prescribe HRT for a limited amount of time, anyway, meaning that even if HRT helps you, your symptoms may return after you stop using it. Once again, you and your doctor should consider whether this is the right path for you.

Such interventions don't really address the underlying change that is menopause. Menopause, with its myriad changes to all parts of you — mind, body, and heart — has a message for you: If you've been neglecting your needs in order to satisfy the wants and needs of everyone else, now it's time for you to take center stage in your own life.

Many women get used to counting on their bodies, hearts, and minds to just "do their jobs" while they raise their families and build their careers. I know I did. I expected to be able to do what I needed to do in order to support my child and work my job, but with minimal support of my body. I expected to be able to remain relatively even-handed emotionally. I depended on my ability to multitask and juggle home, work, and community responsibilities.

Okay, I wasn't in great shape physically. And my personal life wasn't nearly as satisfying as I'd once hoped it would be. But I was an adult. I was a wife and a mother and a systems analyst with a lot of responsibility at work. I also volunteered for good causes. Those are the important things to prioritize when you're an adult, right?

Except.

Except for that nagging discontent that caught up with me when I was in my late forties. I had a sense that my wants and needs were somehow considered less important than anyone else's. Not only did everyone else consider my wants and needs less important, I'd also bought into that way of thinking.

The changes that happen during menopause are often the catalyst that helps us realize we're important, too. This happens, in part, because our health feels compromised and so we take more notice of our bodies. All the changes in our bodies that come during the process of going through menopause may help us pay attention to and attempt to improve our health.

The changes in the way you think and feel may be a signal that it's time to rebalance more than just your hormones. Those changes may be telling you it's time to rebalance your life, with your own needs more prominently featured. Not by dumping your responsibilities (although you may want to give some away), but by adding your own health — your physical, mental, and emotional needs — into the mix of what you give your attention to.

In the next few chapters, I'll tell you about some of the ways you can begin to recapture your health — and yourself.

# CHAPTER 5

# SPEAKING OF FOOD...

The generations of women going through menopause right now — the last of the baby boomers and the first of Generation X — are unlike those who came before us. We're the first generations to be brought up in houses where televisions were the norm and convenience foods had begun to replace meals made from primary ingredients. We were the first to eat fast food and the first for whom restaurant meals were normal. These firsts are not special in a good way.

We were also the first generations to be taught about the "food pyramid" in elementary school. We were the first to have large amounts of genetically modified organisms (GMOs) in our food (even though that didn't happen until we were older). And we were the first for whom chemical preservatives in our food became a way of life.

The first to live with vaccines and antibiotics our whole lives.

The first for whom office jobs — jobs where sitting all day is the norm — have been more prevalent (and considered more desirable!) than physical labor. The first generations raised with "rush hour" and "gridlock."

Now, don't get me wrong — I'm not going to go all "everything new or scientific is wrong" on you. But those things

I listed have changed the way we live, how we age, and how we go through menopause.

Some of the changes *are* good. Vaccines for polio, measles, smallpox, diphtheria, and so many more diseases have saved countless lives. I'm not sure I'd want to live anymore in a world without computers and electronic communication (even if I'd like to take a weekend off now and then). When I was younger, I sure wouldn't have been happy living without tampons! And we live in a kinder and gentler world than the one my parents grew up in.

But some of these changes are not so good. We're only now learning how careful we need to be when we change our food supply and the way we eat. And the way we move our bodies. And the way we approach our health.

I certainly don't want to go back to that previous way of living. But when our bodies are stressed by hormonal changes, as they are when we're going through perimenopause and postmenopause, we're more vulnerable to factors that compound our health risks. Factors like a careless diet, a sedentary lifestyle, stress levels that stay elevated for months (or years!), and not having the support we need can make it harder to get through menopause.

We need a supportive, healthy environment more than ever before.

I see our health as being supported by four pillars: nutrition, movement, stress management, and the support we need. And that's what we're going to examine in this book. I'm going to give you my best advice, the advice I share with my private clients, to bring your hormones into the best possible balance, to help you get to an optimal state of health, and to prepare the way for you to live your best life ever.

## A WORD ABOUT WEIGHT

I know that many of you are looking for a solution to help you lose weight. I admit that was my own road that led me to the discovery of most of the information in this book. Weight loss was what got me interested in how menopause affects us. I wanted to figure out how to be at a body weight and size that felt good. That I could brag about, even.

But, along the way, I discovered a whole lot more. I found out that being healthy was more important than being skinny. That what I really wanted was to be able to do the things I wanted to do. And, even more important than that, I wanted to love the person I was becoming and the life I was creating for myself.

For the most part, those things don't depend on whether you're a size two or a size 12 or a size 22. I've seen women be happy and healthy at all those sizes — women who love themselves, their bodies, and their lives; who are loved by friends and family; women who are following their passions in the world.

I've also seen unhealthy, unhappy women at all those sizes — women who didn't treat themselves with love, but instead berated themselves for what they were or weren't; women who couldn't believe that they could choose to live with joy, health, and passion.

If you want to lose weight and your weight is in the way of you being healthy and happy, I really want to help with that. But if, for you, you're here for symptom relief, wanting glowing health and happiness at whatever weight, this information is for you, too. Because this is all about being your best you — no matter what menopause throws your way!

## NUTRITION — HOW WE EAT

Getting healthy begins with food. That's not a new concept. It's been part of our cultural knowledge for more than 24 centuries. That's when Hippocrates said, "Let food be thy medicine and medicine be thy food." He knew that eating a diet that's high in the right stuff and low in the wrong stuff promotes health. But now we've gotten stuck in a world where we don't even know what a healthy diet looks like. Or, at least, it seems to take a lot of effort to figure out what we need to do to support our bodies through menopause.

Although the "healthy diet" in America has taken a few weird turns in the past 50 years, we're starting to get a handle by now on what really works for health. We're even starting to understand how menopausal hormone imbalances and all the other hormone imbalances are affected by what we eat. This information is really new. It's only been around for the past two or three years!

I'd like to tell you what led me to figuring this whole thing out. I didn't start out with a background in nutrition or medicine. I was like you — entering perimenopause with *no* idea of what to expect. My eating habits weren't based on anything other than eating what I liked: sugary things, bread, fried foods. Yeah, the worst of the Standard American Diet (SAD).

I ate doughnuts for breakfast, pizza for lunch, and for dinner I ate at whatever restaurant caught my fancy. I admit to never having been skinny, but I'd always been able to do what I wanted to do, physically. As I entered perimenopause, it became harder to stay active and to be active when I wanted to be. As my marriage fell apart, I kept gaining weight. And there were symptoms I was having that I wasn't even recognizing yet.

Something had to give. Or, more accurately, I had to give something up. I had to give up eating whatever I wanted. Give up pretending it didn't matter that I was unhappy with my body. Give up thinking that my health didn't matter.

After my marriage ended, I made a decision. I decided that I could either let that failure kill me or I could make it the best thing that had ever happened to me. I began by focusing on weight loss. In the more than ten years since then, I've learned a lot. And I now realize that maybe weight loss isn't the best first step.

But, hey, it's what got me here, and if it's what gets you started, then use that motivation!

## WHAT ARE THE RIGHT FOODS?

Let's talk about what makes eating "right" in midlife.

We all know what the right foods are, don't we? Aren't they the ones on that food pyramid we learned about back in fourth grade? Grains are at the bottom of the pyramid — eat the most of them, six to eleven servings a day; fruits and vegetables, five to nine servings; dairy, two to three servings; and meats (and other proteins), two to three servings. Eat fats, oils, and sweets "sparingly." That's what I remember about the food pyramid from grade school, and I'll bet you learned something similar.

And then there was the low-fat trend — fueled by research that said all cholesterol was bad for the heart and by the "common sense" notion that *eating* fat must contribute to *being* fat. Thus the campaign to eliminate fat from food. Except that everything then tasted so much like cardboard that they added sugar. Lots of sugar.

Until lately. Until the research sparked by the low-carb diets of Dr. Atkins, Dr. Sears, and half a dozen others started showing up in mainstream medical and science journals. Now food is allowed to taste good again — without the addition of sugar or high-fructose corn syrup; without removing the fat; without eliminating meat or egg yolks!

Why? Because now we know that *eating* fats doesn't cause you to *get* fat. And we know that dietary cholesterol doesn't contribute to blood serum cholesterol, for most people. Okay, let's be real here. Sure, if you drink a bottle of olive oil, you're gonna gain some weight. And if you weigh 300 pounds, you're probably gonna have cholesterol issues. And overeating combined with a sedentary lifestyle *are* real health issues. But our understanding of cause and effect has shifted.

What does today's "right" healthy diet include? Let's take a look.

**Protein.** Current recommendations for protein include up to 35 percent of calories from protein. Protein comes from meat, fish, dairy, eggs, nuts, seeds, and a variety of grain and legume sources. Grains aren't always the best choice, but they are important protein sources for many vegetarians, so if you don't eat meat, you may need to keep them in your diet.

**Non-Starchy Vegetables.** Almost all the foods that we consider vegetables (yeah, a tomato's a fruit — I know, but I am talking about the foods we commonly think of as vegetables, like tomatoes) are great, healthy food. They're low in calories, high in fiber, and have lots of important vitamins and minerals, including trace elements you won't get from a Flintstones chewable. Plus, they taste amazing, especially when they're fresh. And they fill you up.

**Fats.** You need fat in your diet. Up to about 30 to 35 percent of your calories are recommended to come from fat. *But* it needs to be healthy fat. Unfortunately, this is where the science of the 1930s, 1940s, and 1950s really screwed up. When nutritionists started admitting that trans fats and vegetable oils weren't healthier than saturated fats, I remember my mom saying, "But they *told* us margarine was better than butter." In fact, trans fats like those found in margarine are just plain deadly. So, what are the best fats? Olive oil and coconut oil, along with nut and seed oils, like walnut and flaxseed oil. Saturated fats are no longer the enemy, either, so go ahead and enjoy those more fatty cuts of meat and don't banish the egg yolks — that's where the nutrition is.

Then there are the things you really, really shouldn't eat. Ever. Even if they taste like the best stuff. The good news is that there are only a few of these, and the ones you're afraid I'm going to put on this list aren't there. There's good science behind each of these exclusions from the "right" food list. (My ISG — Inner Science Geek — has put all that science stuff on my website here: www.menopause. guru/misg/category/food).

Here are the things to really avoid:

**High fructose corn syrup (HFCS).** My ISG has a *lot* to say about this garbage. It's bad for you and it's everywhere. High-fructose corn syrup is *not* the same as sugar, no matter what the corn producers want you to believe. Avoid it!

**Artificial Sweeteners.** Avoid them (except stevia — the jury's still out on this one). These are manufactured chemicals, and some people have extreme sensitivities to them. There's no good reason to use artificial sweeteners in foods and no good will come of eating them.

**Trans fats.** These are chemically-modified fats, which have been altered to extend shelf life. They're found in many processed foods, like deep-fried foods, baked goods, snack foods, and margarine. Even the Food and Drug Administration (FDA) says there's no safe amount of trans fats to eat, except for naturally occurring ones, which mostly enter our diet from certain meats. You'll often find these fats listed in food ingredient lists and on food labels as "partially hydrogenated oil" or "hydrogenated vegetable oil."

**Chemical preservatives, artificial flavors, and ingredients with long, complicated chemical names.** Just say no to artificial food! This includes MSG. And nitrites and sulfites, both of which are found in lunch meats and bacon — although there are some lunch meats and bacon out there that don't have artificial additives.

That's it! Only four things to really avoid. Of course, doing so leaves almost all processed and pre-packaged foods out of your diet.

You might have thought I was going to include alcohol and caffeine in that no-good list. Or that I was going to urge you to give up sugar and flour and oatmeal and a whole bunch of stuff you're in love with. Nope! You can eat everything that's on the good list in the previous section, in reasonable quantities. But anything on the bad list? Avoid it like the food plague it is.

What about foods that aren't covered in either list, like grains, alcohol, and even sugar? Well, then it depends. It depends on *you*. On whether your hormones need certain kinds of dietary support or are hoping you'll avoid certain foods. On whether you have a food sensitivity. On whether you're trying to lose weight. That's why your diet is such a personal choice!

Let's talk now about making those food choices, by looking at some common situations and taking hormone issues into consideration.

**What if adrenal fatigue is kicking my butt?** It's not uncommon for women in any of the stages of menopause to find that their cortisol level is extremely high or that their adrenal glands aren't working right and their cortisol levels are too low. Just to recap from Chapter Three, when you've been under stress for an extraordinary amount of time, your adrenal glands fatigue and no longer pump out enough of any of the hormones they produce. Even though your body is trying to produce a high amount of cortisol, it can't, and your cortisol levels appear low. From a dietary standpoint, high cortisol and low cortisol get treated the same way. You've got to forget about weight loss for the short term, because you're in a fairly serious state and your health is at risk.

This is the one time when carbs (whole grains, legumes, beans, starchy vegetables, and a higher daily portion of fruit) are a vital part of your diet. Your body needs energy in order to mend. It needs to relax, and you need to help it sense that all is right with the world so that the need for cortisol production will decrease. Enjoy adequate portions of any foods (except the four types of food to avoid). Consider avoiding alcohol and caffeine, as they can both stress your adrenals — but only if doing so won't create a physical withdrawal problem. Refined grains and sugars are still best kept at low levels even if you're going through adrenal fatigue.

**What if I'm stress-eating?** Stress-eating often involves comfort foods. For me, that's a grilled cheese sandwich on white bread with applesauce and sweet pickles on the side. That's what I want when I have the flu or when I miss my mom and dad. Is it okay to eat comfort food when you're craving it? Well, yes. Occasionally. And if you can avoid continuing to do it for too long. How do you keep from eating comfort food for too long? Here's how I handle it: I don't keep the stuff for making comfort food (the ingredients I know aren't the best for me to eat) in the house — because then stress-eating would become a way of life for me! If I need it badly, I go out and buy the stuff (or send my husband, if I have the flu). I've been known to throw out the rest of a loaf of white bread or other items left over after I've had my indulgence.

**What if I'm insulin resistant?** If you're insulin resistant or have been diagnosed with metabolic syndrome or Type 2 Diabetes, ditch any and all grains, minimize beans and legumes, and cut out all sugars, which include many types of fruit, most starchy vegetables, and things like honey, maple syrup, and high fructose corn syrup (HFCS), because those are like poisons for you. This is also the way to go if you can be categorized as morbidly obese (I really hate that official term!), which is often a signal that insulin resistance is just around the corner. (If you've been categorized as morbidly obese, but have had insulin testing done and your blood sugar levels are acceptable, I still recommend making eating a bit of sugar a special treat only). Fruits and starchy vegetables should also be approached with caution. The glycemic index is your friend. This index is a system you can use to help you understand the impact of foods on your blood sugar. If the glycemic index of a food is high (like for bananas, watermelon, and white potatoes), avoid it. If it's low, you can eat that food in moderation. It's easy to find the glycemic index or the index's rating of specific foods — just google *glycemic index* or google the food you're interested in plus *glycemic index*.

**What if I have low metabolism because of my lifestyle or yo-yo dieting?** If your thyroid isn't doing its job of stoking your metabolism, then you'll want to eat and exercise specifically to reset it. For most women, a daily diet of 1500 to 1800 calories of good foods shouldn't cause weight gain. If it does, and your thyroid levels are okay, then consider a plan for metabolic reset. There are several good plans for doing this that I use and that I recommend to my clients, depending on their eating preferences. Each of the different metabolic reset plans calls for eating specific combinations of foods. You can find a list of my favorite metabolic reset diets on my website at www.menopause.guru/wl-plans. (I keep the list on the website, because it's changing all the time, either through new nutritional discoveries or through trying different diets.)

**What if I'm suffering the effects of estrogen dominance?** If you're in early perimenopause and are suffering the effects of estrogen dominance, one solution may be to reduce your intake of grain-fed meat, alcohol, and non-organic produce. Our Western culture's typical meat production processes result in standard (non-organic) meat that raises our estrogen levels, especially our xenoestrogen levels — these are pseudo-estrogens that act like estrogen in bad ways, without giving us any of the positives. Plant crops that are high in pesticides and phytoestrogens, like soy and hops, also contribute to the problem of estrogen dominance.

**What if it's time to party?** Yes, there are times in our lives when we need to take a break and enjoy ourselves. Sometimes, that involves food — holidays, birthdays, celebrations. And sometimes, it's just easier to go with the flow at someone else's house. Yes, it's okay to indulge. But know how to stop after you've indulged or just don't do it in the first place.

I talked with a new client recently who told me she was a world champion at losing five pounds. She's done it over and over. Unfortunately, whenever she reached five pounds, she celebrated. And then she'd "forget" to go back on her diet. By the time we met, the amount of weight she needed to lose wasn't five or seven or even ten pounds, but more like 25.

Most foods are okay, in moderation, or once in a while, or okay for certain people at certain times. The rest of the time, eat what's going to support your health and do your body the most good.

## HOW YOU EAT

There are hundreds of diets out there. Every week, I get about half a dozen notices for new diets in my email. When I go to the bookstore (a particular hobby of mine), I'll see four or five new books about diets and dieting, often by an author who recommended something completely different last year.

So, what makes a diet good for you, and how do you choose which one is best for you?

I don't think there is only one diet that works. I believe the best diet is the one that works for you and that you'll stick with. That means you're happy eating that way *most* of the time. When I help my clients think through their diet preferences and choices, they begin by taking my Personal Dimensions of Diet Assessment, which we go through together.

I've identified five dimensions, corresponding to D-I-E-T-S:

**D** — diversity — how much change from day to day you like in your diet?

**I** — incremental — do you like to "jump in with both feet, or make one change at a time?

**E** — ease — do you need a diet that's fast and easy, or do you like to spend time in the kitchen?

**T** — timing — do you like to eat lots of small meals, or does it feel better to eat less often?

**S** — scoring — are you a person who likes to journal, weigh frequently and "keep score?" Or would you rather just follow the rules and see the results at the end?

All of these factors contribute to how well you'll do with a particular style of eating, or whether you need to modify it to suit your personal preferences. The best diet in the world won't help you weigh less or be healthier if you don't follow it. This exercise helps you figure out how you can create or modify a diet just for you.

One of my clients, Linda, was a busy mother of four, including a teenager and a young woman planning her wedding. Linda had a high-stress job and was heavily committed to volunteer activities. She wanted to lose weight for her daughter's wedding, and was willing to make the changes, but needed a plan simple enough to wedge into her busy life. In order to meet her needs, I analyzed all her preferences and created a plan based on them and on her nutritional needs, so as to support her in the high-stress environment she found herself in. On that plan and with her exercise program, she lost two dress sizes and looked fabulous at her daughter's wedding.

I've made the Personal Dimensions of Diet Assessment available to you. You can take the assessment and get your answers at www.menopause.guru/PDD. Then you can analyze how *you* relate to food, what your best plan looks like, and choose a diet that will work best for you. I've rated my favorite diets at www.menopause.guru/wl-plans according to each of the DIETS scales.

## A FEW LAST RULES

Choosing what to eat is not all about personal preferences. There *are* some rules. Most of the rules are going to be ones that work for you, because they'll be coming from the diet you've selected. But some rules are simply unbreakable. If the diet you've selected asks you to break any of the rules below more than only a little bit, I urge you to question whether it's really a healthy diet.

I advise all my clients to follow these rules. When we work together to select a diet that's a good fit for them, we always check it against these rules. If the diet doesn't follow these rules, I recommend selecting a different one.

1. **You need a minimum number of calories per day.** For almost every woman, the minimum daily calorie intake will be right around 1200. If you're extremely petite, *your doctor* — that's your very own doctor, not the doctor who wrote the diet book — may recommend a lower level. This minimum calorie intake provides the starter fuel you need in order to remain active and to burn additional calories. (In my experience, everyone has a day now and then when eating enough is almost impossible and 1200 calories doesn't happen. That's okay, as long as eating less than 1200 is *not* your daily target.) If you are extremely heavy, your minimum calorie intake could be significantly more. Calculators available online will help you determine what this minimum level should be.

2. **Hydration is crucial.** Adequate water intake is essential. A certain amount of the liquid you consume should be water — not soft drinks or coffee or tea. That's because anything added to water puts stress on your kidneys (and sometimes your liver, too) during its processing, which makes those organs less effective at their job of filtering your blood. Aim for 64 ounces

(eight cups) of liquid a day, with two-thirds of that being plain water. Once that's comfortable, move up to drinking half your body weight in ounces (for example, if you weigh 180 pounds, you'd aim to drink 90 ounces).

3. **Focus on feeling healthy and energetic.** If, after the first couple of weeks on a new eating plan, you feel lousy, sluggish, or overly hyper, consider ditching that plan and finding a new way of eating. Yes, you can feel awful as your body detoxifies and as it changes over to new energy sources, but you should start feeling better within two to three weeks, often sooner.

4. **Focus on whole foods versus chemicals.** Much of our food supply is heavily treated with chemicals. Artificial chemicals are used as everything from preservatives to flavors, and for altering textures and colors. Our meat and dairy products are laced with hormones, and our fruits and vegetables contain pesticides. The effects of some of these additives and pesticides are well-known. Others are in our food, but their effects have barely been explored by research. So eat the most whole and natural form of food, and the highest quality (like organic), that you can manage.

5. **Eat mostly from the "good" foods list above**.

Your diet is going to be all about you and where you are right now. You have unique goals and unique requirements based on the state of your hormonal balance right now. But that can change, both as you fix imbalances and as you continue to go through the process of menopause. So your diet will likely need to be modified at some point, and more than once, to maintain its rightness for you. Even with other factors being equal, as you become

healthier or lose the weight you want to lose, what will work for the next stage of your journey may not be what works for this stage.

This is why I help all of my clients personalize their diets over time — so that their diet stays current as they change. Then they feel good and have a diet plan that works not only today but down the road.

# CHAPTER 6

# JOY IN MOVEMENT

Fair warning: This is my favorite part of the book, so if my enthusiasm for moving my body, for being out and active in the world, gets on your nerves a little, well, I'm not really sorry.

I wasn't always this way. I always have enjoyed some sports, even though I was never very good at any of them. But were they a central part of my being? No, not until I was in my late forties.

At the same time I became serious about changing my life through changing my weight, I realized (mostly because my support team pounded it into me) that I would have to either get at least *some* exercise on a daily basis or face my team's never-ending criticism for getting skinny without getting healthy. The people on my support team appealed to my need for results by convincing me that moving would help me achieve the result I wanted most: weight loss. With my penchant for researching everything, I soon realized they were right.

Even though my goal was weight loss, I wasn't totally oblivious about my health. In fact, one of my main motivations for weight loss was watching a co-worker become increasingly disabled due to weight. Everything from walking up a set of stairs to simply breathing became difficult for her.

That was really scary!

When I started getting daily exercise, I was in the worst shape of my life. I'd been through everything from an illness the previous summer, to no activity over the winter, to trying to eat myself to death as my marriage failed, and all of that had left me at the point where I got winded walking to the mailbox. I told myself that with my schedule — I traveled constantly for work — I didn't have much time for exercise.

I decided to start with walking, because it was easy. At first, my goals were simple. I walked a few minutes on flat terrain. Then I walked a little more each day. I started to get to the point where I wasn't as winded, and I began to notice what was going on around me. I started picking where I walked more carefully, opting for the most beautiful places for watching sunrises and sunsets, the places where the birds would be singing, the reflection of light on water.

It really didn't take long. Within a couple of months, I was walking 40 minutes at a time and actually having trouble doing a walk that was what I thought of as "hard enough." I was eager for results by then. They couldn't come fast enough for me!

So I made a fateful decision. Spurred on by one of my support team members, I looked up a simple running program online. I must have tried running 15 or 20 times in my life before that, and I'd *never* succeeded. Yes, I made every mistake in the book and invented a few new ones on my way to actually accomplishing my fitness goals. But, this time, I discovered the secret to success (psst — it's going *very, very* slowly!).

*Slowly*, over the next few months, I became hooked on running. It took me more than five months to build up to running five kilometers, but then my online support group met in person in Tennessee to do a 5k together, and I ran the whole way!

Running became an anchor for me. Even when the desire to sit and do nothing became strong, my habit of running was stronger.

Being able to run became a lure. If I could change enough to become a runner, what else could I do? It became the lure that led me into the gym, onto a mountain bike, down rivers in kayaks, underwater with scuba tanks. Being able to run led me to health and my best body ever.

Running may not be *your* joy or your destiny. I admit that it's not for everybody. And I'm not even suggesting that you try it. Whatever type of exercise you explore and choose, it's finding *your* body's way of experiencing joy in moving that will make a huge difference in your life.

## WHY MOVE?

What's so important about moving, anyway? Why should you do it?

Maybe at this stage of your life, it seems like so much is in the way of taking time for deliberate movement. There's that "selfish" thing: How do you take time for yourself when there's so much other stuff to do? How do you exercise when you already feel fatigued — whether from not being able to sleep or from sleeping but still waking up tired? Then there are the aches and pains of what feels like having done too much living. And maybe there's a "don't care anymore" feeling.

Are you feeling any of those? Or maybe all of them? Maybe you have a different reason for not wanting to exercise. Maybe you're already convinced you "have to," but you don't know how to start.

I've come to the point where I tend not to talk about "exercise" with my clients. Because "exercise" and "working out" are *work*, right? And work is just more stress. Instead, we talk about finding the joy in moving, making moving fun and feeling good about it. Feeling powerful and taking charge. Doing something good for yourself and enjoying doing it.

For most of us, moving will produce health results faster than changing our eating. Within a few days, you'll be able to walk farther or climb stairs easier or carry an extra bag of groceries into the house. You'll feel more balanced and capable. You may notice a pleasing feeling of hunger before a meal, the sensation that you've earned your meal, instead of that gnawing, "Feed me!" hunger.

All of these tell you you've done it! You've cared for yourself. You've taken action to make yourself healthier and happier. You've accomplished a goal that you set — even if you or someone else thinks that goal is so tiny as to be insignificant. After all, can't every normal person walk to the mailbox? Well, if *you* couldn't or didn't, then *celebrate* that you're doing it today!

## SIDE EFFECTS OF MOVING

Women often bemoan the potential risks and side effects of the drugs they're prescribed for various conditions that overtake them in midlife. Drugs with significant risks include not only hormone replacement therapy treatment, but prescriptions that address high blood pressure, high cholesterol, insulin resistance, depression, anxiety... the list goes on and on. It seems that once you hit midlife, if you go to the doctor, you're likely to find yourself on a drug your doctor wants you to be on for the rest of your life.

Reading the little pamphlet that comes in the box with the drug can be really scary! But, hey, no worries, right? If you experience side effects, the doc will prescribe something for *that*, too.

Well, here's the thing about moving your body: You'll *love* the side effects, like these:

- Better sleep

- Weight loss

- Healthy food tastes better

- Lowered blood pressure and cholesterol

- Reduced anxiety

- Better moods (moving lifts depression and, in general, helps you feel better)

- Better bone strength, better balance, and less risk of falling

- Better muscle tone (smaller clothing size)

- Better skin, hair, and nails

- Better hormonal balance

Those are only a few of the ways that making moving a part of your daily life improves your quality of life. I bet if you give moving a try for a month, you'll have an expanded list of positive side effects of your own!

## HOW DO YOU MAKE MOVING FUN?

Maybe I've convinced you that there's a benefit to getting moving, but you're still not ready to head to the nearest gym and put your body out there in front of all those body-builders and gym rats, or to trip over your feet in a Zumba class, or join the local running club. I get it. It took me a long time to build up the confidence (and the skill) to try those things (and I'm still not sure about Zumba!).

Yep, exercise is hard, sweaty, and boring. Workouts are *work*, even when we call them "finding the joy in moving." But there are endless varieties of ways to move and enjoy it, without even setting foot in a gym, and this means you can find a way to feel the joy of moving, too.

When helping people find a way to move that feels more like joy than work, I like to start with asking the question, "What was fun for you when you were a kid? Or a teenager? Or a young woman?" Even as a bookish, nerd-kid, I liked being in the woods, and I liked climbing trees. I wasn't much for team sports, but I could ride my bike for hours. Is it any wonder that I now love to go mountain biking?

What was your way of moving when you were a kid? Did you go for the solo activities? Or did you prefer a team sport? Dancing with your girlfriends (or boyfriends)? Did you like to go roller skating on Friday nights? Bowling? Did you enjoy being outside?

These are all clues to the types of activities you might like to choose now. The really cool thing about the world we live in now is that so many options are available to us, from riding a bike on a converted railroad bed to playing "soccer" while encased in a giant bubble. You can find or make your own fun in dozens and dozens of ways. Don't believe me? Just think of something you might like and Google it. Find something that looks like fun and make it your goal to try it out, move your body, make it happen.

## HOW DO YOU START?

Let's say you're like Marcia. Marcia really wanted to be a runner. She had been a runner back in high school when she ran track. When we talked about what she wanted to do to move her body, it was run a 5k. But because she hadn't been exercising for so long and was out of shape, she was frustrated. She couldn't even run a block, much less a 5k! She was ready to give up before she'd even started.

Whenever you start doing any kind of movement, you can't jump ahead. That's a prescription for disaster — injury, frustration, quitting before you get results. Marcia and I worked together to benchmark where she was, to see how close she was to being able to run a 5k, and she realized that she loved to take her infant granddaughter out for long strolls. That was exercise she was already getting.

Because Marcia could walk for 40 minutes without stopping, I invited her to begin her training for a 5k with a running program I modified just for her. I let her know that she'd need to carefully monitor her eating to bring her weight down and keep from endangering her knees. Twelve weeks later, Marcia was registered for that 5k. She laughs and says that she probably could have walked that first 5k faster than she ran it, but nothing can part her from the "participation medal" she got for that 5k.

Marcia reached her goal by starting where she was, not where she used to be, not where she wanted to be, not where her best friend was. She did it by following a proven plan. She did it by not getting impatient and not giving up.

## WHAT IF YOU'RE NOT READY?

It's easy to say you'll start running slowly. I read an article once that suggested that returning runners start slowly and don't run more than a mile their first time out. But what if running one step looks impossible? Or swimming one lap? Or even pushing your grandchild on the swing? What if fibromyalgia or arthritis or another chronic condition makes every movement painful?

When I'm helping a woman who's extremely limited, we always start where she is. When working with Ellen, whose weight had gotten completely out of control, we started with standing for one minute — that was it. A month later, she could walk for five minutes at a time and had lost ten percent of her body weight!

Always begin with what you can do without pain. For Ellen, it was standing. She moved on to being able to walk in place and was eventually able to walk around her block. If you're dealing with fibromyalgia or similar conditions, I know it's hard to believe, but movement will actually make things better, *if* you start slowly.

## IS THERE ANYTHING YOU SHOULD AVOID?

Remember that old saw, "No pain is no gain"? It's right, but change the punctuation: "No, pain is *no* gain!" Sometime, when you start moving you'll feel uncomfortable, both while you're active and afterwards. When I first started walking, my thighs would get itchy, right on the surface. That turns out to be pretty typical, since more blood is reaching the surface and expanding the capillaries for the first time in a long time. It was a very annoying feeling, but it stopped happening after two or three days.

The first few times I walked, I was a bit sore for the next day or two. Even with stretching and being careful as I'd take it up a notch, I'd feel it the next day. As long as it was only sore, no problem. It's when you go beyond discomfort to pain that you want to be careful. Once or twice, I pushed it too hard and was beyond sore. Walking, sitting, climbing the stairs — all were impossible. Instead of achieving my goals faster, by pushing too hard I delayed my progress. Yep, I should have dialed it back sooner!

## WHAT ABOUT HORMONAL ISSUES?

I love moving. I think it can help *almost* everyone. I don't think there are really many bad ways to get active. But when we're dealing with the changes in our hormones, there are better and worse ways to get moving based on where you are right now. So, what's good and bad for what conditions?

**High or low cortisol.** Remember that extremely low cortisol is the aggravation of an extremely stressed state. It's what happens when your adrenal glands begin to not be able to keep up. If you're dealing with adrenal fatigue (or are so stressed it's likely to happen), your choice of exercise must be gentle, stress-free, and leave you feeling more relaxed than when you started.

The problem is that if you're a high-stress person, you may be wanting to do a rigorous workout routine and go on a stringent diet. That would only compound the problem.

If you're dealing with cortisol issues, be gentle with yourself. Fortify yourself with good foods, extra carbohydrates, and limit your exercise to yoga, stretching, and perhaps some gentle walking.

**Insulin resistance.** Insulin resistance occurs when your body's cells don't respond to insulin's request to take in blood sugar. It occurs because there's too much blood sugar circulating. The body's cells don't need the sugar that's there, because they're already full of fuel, and the fuel that's there isn't being used.

Insulin resistance can be the precursor for an extremely dangerous disease, Type 2 Diabetes. However, insulin resistance — even Type 2 Diabetes — is super-responsive to diet and exercise.

If you have insulin resistance, then vigorous exercise — cardio and weight-bearing (and muscle-building) exercise — will begin to reprogram your body's cells to use the circulating blood sugar. By combining this type of exercise with an extremely low carbohydrate diet, insulin resistance disappears in short order. If you continue this type of plan, the need for medications goes away. Yes, Type 2 Diabetes can be cured through diet and exercise. It just takes consistency!

**Slow metabolism.** What some might think is a thyroid condition is actually a slow metabolism, exercise can be extremely helpful in restarting metabolism. This type of low metabolism is a frequent effect of yo-yo dieting (continuous fluctuations in weight) or extremely low calorie dieting.

The most effective type of exercise to help correct a slow metabolism is very intense, short bursts of exercise. Some helpful exercise methods for this condition are Tabata, HIIT (High-Intensity Interval Training), circuit training, and METabata. What you're looking for is anything that combines short intervals of intense exercising, either cardio or with weights, with very short intervals of rest (a typical ratio for experienced exercisers would be 50 seconds of work followed by ten seconds of rest).

When using one of these exercise protocols, make sure to perform the work interval at an intensity that is hard for you, but not impossible. Remember that "No, pain is *no* gain?" It applies here, too.

**Testosterone imbalances.** Even though testosterone and other androgens can help you feel great, when they get out of balance on the high side, they can create a number of annoying symptoms (including male-pattern baldness, chin hairs, and acne). Exercise for high testosterone imbalance includes moderate-intensity cardio, especially for longer periods of time. Low testosterone imbalance can be helped by weight-lifting (though you don't have to grunt!). Heavy weights, low reps, and long rest intervals seems to be the best protocol for raising testosterone and the other androgens.

**Estrogen imbalances.** Moderate exercise appears to lower out-of-control estrogen, which can cause estrogen dominance. Although after menopause, moderate exercise may reduce levels of estrogen to some extent, the overall health benefits of an active lifestyle outweigh any reduction in estrogen — especially since estrogen appears to be what feeds breast cancer, among other things. The benefits of exercise, like increased muscle and strengthened bones, counter some of the effects of lowered estrogen.

* * *

There are plenty of nuances with these recommendations. It's not unusual to have two or more imbalances at the same time. That means you might have to decide which condition to address first when you're creating your plan. This may mean figuring out a detailed plan that matches your imbalances with a food plan and a movement plan that will correct first one, then another imbalance. Improved health is the result!


## WHY GO ADVENTURING?

One last topic about movement. When I speak to groups of women, I often talk about my adventures. You see, not only did I get hooked on moving — running, biking, dancing — I also got hooked on adventuring — going on out and doing stuff that's, frankly, a bit scary.

Some of the adventurous things I do are only scary in the thinking about it. Yes, I've jumped out of a perfectly good airplane. And, yes, it was terrifying. That is, until I started floating down to earth. Then (and I know you may not believe me), it was about as much fun as one person can have with another person strapped on their back (okay, ladies, keep it clean!).

I encourage you to do something that scares you. Why? Because when you step out and do something you're afraid of, you realize that courage isn't not being afraid — it's not letting fear stop you. We're all afraid from time to time.

We're unsure about the consequences of an action we'd like to take. We're scared to step into the full power of our dreams.

But, guess what? When you *do* step up and have an adventure, you discover how powerful you are. You find out that you *can* change your world from one where "I couldn't possibly do that" to one where "Yep! That's done!" And once you've done something, it's never closed off to you again.

Also, when I go adventuring (and drag others along with me), I find myself out in the great, wide, beautiful world, and I'm reminded of just how beautiful it is.

Yes, fulfilling your dreams can be scary, but once you've gone adventuring, you have that experience as a memory that helps you remember how courageous you are. The fear itself might not go away as you continue to have adventures, but you realize that fear can't make you stop going after your dreams.

Finally, go adventuring because it's *fun*, and you deserve to have fun! You deserve pleasure, whether from riding down a water slide, going kayaking on a bayou, or steering a mountain bike down a bumpy trail. Or maybe your version of adventuring is stretching yourself by taking a photography workshop (or being the model). Maybe adventure, to you, means taking a trip by yourself.

Moving and adventure are fun. You'll see. And *you* are entitled to fun. You really are!

## JUST KEEP MOVING!

Movement can be a hard habit to build. There's plenty that would like to get in your way. There are always other things you could be doing instead. There are often sore muscles. There's hot weather or cold weather, rain or snow. There's fear, and there's simply not wanting to move.

Don't let any of that stop you. Don't let *anything* stop you. Because, I promise, once moving becomes a habit, you'll wonder why it took you so long to do this for yourself.

# CHAPTER 7

# JUST *RELAX*!

Okay, I'm ready to agree that there's no stupider topic to bring up with women in any stage of their menopausal journey than stress reduction. There's no stupider advice than, "Just relax! Don't sweat the small stuff! Go with the flow!" Yeah, when you feel like you're on the 58th day of your period or when you've had 92 hot flashes since last night or when your hormones have you so jacked up you're ready to kill your dog (or maybe even your husband), "Go with the flow!" is exactly what you want to hear, right?

So, let me be clear. This chapter is *not* about stress reduction. The sources of stress in your life aren't likely to go away. At least, not without access to a clandestine burial site (a little menopausal humor). You can't ditch your job, your husband, your husband's obnoxious best friend, *your* best friend (who never *used* to be so obnoxious), your kids, your house, your dog, your parents, or, of course, the biggest stressor of all — your body. Those things (and probably a dozen other things stressing you out) are part of your life. And, truth be told, you really do love most of them. Most of the time.

Except maybe your body.

I know — now that I've brought up the topic of stress, you're depressed. When everything was going wrong for me and my stress level was through the roof, I was trying to deal with it by googling "stress reduction," going to yoga classes, and exercising my way through stress, but it always seemed like there was still the same amount of stress in my life!

My ex was still a jerk. My son was still an adrenaline junkie. My pets still wanted more attention from me than I had for them, starting from the moment I walked in the door. Airport security personnel could still be obnoxious. I was having a house built 1300 miles from where I lived (and 2400 miles from where I worked!). The phone would ring and I'd brace myself to go through the roof. Again!

Then, one day, I decided to give massage a try. For a whole hour, not one single thought stayed in my head long enough to create tension. No matter what I thought (yes, the thoughts would appear — I remember that much), they slipped away before I could concentrate on them, before I could get emotional about them, before I could think, "But what if..."

Not long after that, my running (okay, more like a fast shuffle) intervals increased to five or so minutes. As I stopped spending my exercise time checking in with my body parts to make sure they weren't falling off and stopped listening to my labored breathing and stressing over what had gone wrong at work, a new sensation took over. For most of the running interval, I'd simply count my footfalls in my head: "1-and-2-and-3-and-4-and-1-and..." round and round. Thoughts that had been plaguing me disappeared in the calming routine of the count.

Soon, I began seeking that sensation of letting go of my thoughts, letting them pass on through. I began to realize that there were other times and places for thinking those thoughts, gnawing on those worries, and I could have a break from them. I found times and spaces in which to open up to the sensation of just being.

Finding those more peaceful spaces didn't make the stressors go away. It didn't make my ex less of a jerk. It didn't stop my son from taking crazy risks, or my mother from being controlling. It didn't mean I had fewer problems with the house contractor, or that it was any easier commuting from New Hampshire to California for work. It *did* mean that finding times to step away from the stressors helped me look at situations a little more objectively. I began to realize that sometimes I could choose my reaction to a stressor.

That's what we're looking into in this chapter: ways of toning down the stress until it's at a level you feel comfortable enough with to choose your reactions.

## WHY STRESS IS AN IMPORTANT TOPIC

Stress is a common theme during menopause. We talked about the stress hormone cortisol and how the way it operates in our bodies changes as our estrogen levels change. We talked about how anxiety and panic attacks are common symptoms of perimenopause and menopause. We talked about how adrenal fatigue is the result when our bodies can no longer keep up the demand for cortisol production.

What we haven't really talked about is what those elevated levels of cortisol and feelings of stress do to us. Yes, they can create panic attacks. Yes, we feel overwhelmed. But there's more to it than that. Remember I said that we weren't designed to be under constant stress? We're designed for the quick attack and resolution. Let's look more closely at how that works (Inner Science Geek alert!).

In the moment of panic (when the snake slithers across your path, if you have a near-accident on the highway, when the phone rings at 2 a.m.), here's what happens: Your perceptive systems signal your adrenal glands to release cortisol and epinephrine. These trigger a rise in heart rate, respiration rate, and blood pressure. Your body gets ready to respond to danger. Your muscles tense and blood is shunted away from digestion to your muscles and your brain — but not to the thinking part of your brain (the neocortex). The danger signal turns up the dial on your senses, making you feel hyperaware, and gets you ready to fight or flee.

The most primitive part of your brain has taken over. This is the *amygdala*, and it's designed to, no matter what, keep you alive. It's the part that gets you to fight or flee. Most of all, it's the part of your brain that resists change at all costs. One name for it is "the lizard brain" (yes, we share this structure with reptiles!), which I've shortened to "Lizzie."

If there's a danger and you and Lizzie take evasive action, then you're safe. Maybe your heart pounds for a few minutes longer, and you may feel tired as the epinephrine (also called adrenaline) leaves your body. But what if the danger — or your sense that there's danger — goes on longer? Maybe you've had an important lab test done and the results aren't going to be back for a few days. Your body could experience short-term stress effects.

You may not experience all of the stress effects I list below, or for all of the time, as you wait for those test results to come back, but if something reminds you about the test, if you check your phone for messages about the test, if someone asks you about the test, the stress feelings and reactions may return full force. You sweat; you may have cold hands and feet; you may have digestive reactions like nausea, vomiting, or diarrhea; your muscles may become sore from the tension; you may not be able to think straight about complex problems. Since your heart rate and breathing are high, you may experience the feeling of anxiety or panic. You look for instant relief from the stress and may feel frustrated, irritable, or angry when you don't get it.

Let's say the stress keeps on going even further, like for weeks or months, as many of our stressors in the modern world can. Maybe there's a child in trouble in your life, or you're having a work situation that just won't resolve. In such cases, here's what can happen to your body: Your immune system and your libido can both become depressed, because your body deems other systems to be more important. Digestion isn't as important either, so digestive problems become chronic. Ongoing muscle tension creates alignment issues that can result in chronic headaches, backaches, and even joint issues. Your heart can become stressed from running on a continuous "high" setting, and you may notice irregular heartbeats, palpitations, and develop high blood pressure. Your body, fearing imminent famine, stores excess calories and lowers your metabolism, so that you gain weight in your belly.

At this point, you may be wondering if this is *really* how your body reacts, because it sounds pretty awful. Let's try a little experiment. Think of something that would stress you out or scare you (for me, it's that aforementioned snake). Now picture that thing in your mind. Make it as real as you can. Do you feel your breath getting shallower and quicker, your heart beating faster, your muscles tenser? Take a quick survey of your body and notice how even this imaginary stress is affecting you. Feel your stomach muscles clench. Where else are you feeling it? Now imagine this feeling going on and on and on for days. When you're under stress that doesn't let up, this is exactly what happens. It may not be quite this intense, but the effect over time is like water dripping on stone. Sooner or later, no matter how hard the stone, it's going to be changed.

Chronic stress effects aren't just limited to your body. They affect all the rest of you, too — your heart, mind, and spirit.

Emotionally, you may become depressed and feel ineffective, because you can't solve the problem or make it go away. You may withdraw from people you care about and activities you love. You may develop disordered eating — eating too much or not enough (or, even worse, developing bulimia or anorexia).

Mentally, you may lose sharpness, motivation, and focus. You may find yourself stuck in catastrophic thinking (believing that the worst — or way worse than the realistic worst — outcome is probable). You may be easily distracted and quickly slide into worry and anxiety. You may throw yourself into other activities obsessively, to distract yourself from what's causing you stress (computer solitaire, anyone?).

Finally, even the most spiritually grounded person may begin to find themselves losing hope, neglecting to attend to their spiritual life, turning away from their core beliefs and values. That's not a place I want to be, and it's one I hope you never find yourself in.


## HOW DO YOU REDUCE THE STRESS?

Sometimes, trying to deal with stress is like standing against a closed door and pushing on it to hold back the forces that are trying to beat it down. You don't know what's on the other side, but you know you're afraid of it. You can't change what's on the other side, you can only push back against it. It's like living through a bad horror flick!

The thing is, you *don't* know what's on the other side. Yes, whatever it is seems frightening and dangerous, and so you feel like you need to keep that door shut at all costs.

That's how I felt when my whole being started changing with the onset of perimenopause. I didn't know what was happening, only that it didn't feel good and I was scared. I didn't want things to change — not even the things that weren't going well. Because, if things didn't change, I would continue to know what to expect. Even if what was normal for me was uncomfortable, staying the same didn't feel as dangerous as changing.

Using stress management tools to rethink a situation is a lot like starting by putting a peephole or even a window in that door (bulletproof, of course, because I know what *that* horror show music means!). When you start to take away the stress, even a little bit at first, you can begin to calm Lizzie — the fight-or-flight lizard part of your brain — and more of the rest of your brain becomes available again.

Another thing you can do is get curious about what's on the other side of that door. Maybe you can change the soundtrack of your life from horror flick to romantic comedy, or even inspirational, overcome-the-odds film.

When you turn Lizzie and the stress down, you get to *choose* how you're going to perceive and react to the things that are causing you stress.

When it's menopause that's on the other side of the door, turning the stress down can help you begin to realize that menopause may be delivering gifts you never thought you'd get.

## TOOLS FOR TURNING DOWN THE STRESS

I teach a myriad of tools for stress management to the women I work with. I've already shared two of my favorites with you: eating right and moving your body.

Eating right (not stress eating, not choosing crap for the momentary burst of relief) is a big key to supporting yourself when stress is knocking at your door. One thing about stress eating is that it offers a great clue about what you're feeling. If you're likely to reach for the Oreos when stress hits, then doing so is a great indication that stress is around. So pay attention when you find that you've just eaten four Oreos without even knowing where they came from!

Movement is great for reducing stress for a couple of reasons. Both cortisol and epinephrine are "used up" by movement. When you're stressed, you're often itching for action, because that's what those stress hormones are designed to do: get us ready to deal with the threat. Menopause ramps up the way cortisol makes us feel. *Moving* not only stimulates the good neurotransmitters (serotonin and dopamine), it also helps the stress hormones go away. Just the act of doing something — anything — can help you feel like you're taking action to make things better.

When you regularly practice eating right and moving, stress becomes a whole lot easier to manage.

I'll also give you three other tools to help you manage day-to-day stress or a specific stressor. These simple tools work for almost anybody, and they're quick and easy. Their effects may not last long (especially when you're first starting to use them), but you can combine them to give yourself some breathing room when stress threatens to take over.

First things first. Breathe! Draw a breath in, all the way down. Allow your belly to rise — even if you have to undo your belt! Imagine that breath traveling all the way down to your fingers and toes. Then let it out, feeling all the tension leaving with the exhale. Exhale somewhat forcefully, blowing tension away from your body. Breathe in again. Breathe in serenity and calmness. Slow your breathing. Count your breaths, like this: inhale-2-3-4, hold-2-3-4, exhale-2-3-4. After breathing for five or six deep breaths (it will take almost a minute to do that), you should feel tension start to drain away.

The second technique, progressive relaxation, helps with letting go of muscle tension. It's best done either seated or lying down (preferably alone and *never* while driving). Begin with your feet and tense those muscles as hard as you can. Hold for a count of three and then let *all* of the tension go. Move up your body by muscle groups. I usually use this sequence: feet, legs, butt, hands, arms, stomach, chest and back, neck, head and face. What this process helps you do is release tension in muscles you hadn't even realized are tense. Progressive relaxation is really effective when paired with the breathing exercise.

When my thoughts begin flying out of control, I find this third technique of grounding to be particularly helpful. You may have to get creative to find a place to do this one, but it's worth it. Grounding is simply reconnecting with the powerful and nurturing energy of the Earth. Find a small patch of natural ground — ground that supports life. It could be in a park, on a lawn, in a garden, or in the woods. The more you feel connected to nature and life, the better. Beaches or other bodies of water are also good locations for this technique. You can even do this while standing in the water.

This technique is not complicated: Take off your shoes and socks and simply stand on the ground in your bare feet.

Feel the ground beneath your feet. Tune in to the fact that it is nurturing you, as the Earth nourishes all things. You can dig your toes in. You can sit or lie on the ground. Feel your connection with the world, realize that you're part of a whole, yet also complete in yourself. Breathe. Connect to what's divine and what's divine in you, however you conceive of that.

You can do all three of these techniques together. As you do, I hope you begin to feel a difference.

## BEYOND STRESS

In the previous two chapters, we've talked about cortisol, the stress hormone. This chapter is about some of the dangers of not dealing with your stress levels, and how to begin to reduce them.

When you begin to remove the effects of stress, your view of your life may change. You may see the benefits of the changes you've decided to make. You may feel more optimistic about things working out. You may feel great and expect to continue to feel great. Most of all, though, you'll know that if you start getting stressed again, you have tools to use to stop it before it becomes overwhelming!

# CHAPTER 8

# LISTENING TO THE MESSAGES

Where do our symptoms come from? Why does one person seem to have every symptom on the list, and the next person only a few intense symptoms, and the next person almost no symptoms at all? Why do so many doctors think that menopause symptoms are all in our heads and go on to prescribe anti-depressants and anti-anxiety drugs at least as often as hormone replacement therapy (HRT)? Why do some women's symptoms appear long before tests show hormonal levels consistent with perimenopause?

Why do some women do "everything right" (diet, exercise, supplements, and more) and still have symptoms that don't quit? One symptom goes away, but then another one appears. And why does another woman do everything "wrong," but breezes through perimenopause with barely a single night sweat?

Let's get one thing straight before I go any further. I would *never* suggest that any symptom you have is "all in your head." There are definitely things you can do to change the way your symptoms affect you — starting with nutrition, exercise, and stress management. But, I think there's often more to it than that.

My belief is that our bodies, hearts, minds, and, yes, our spirits are linked together in ways that modern medicine is only now beginning to understand*. This means that during menopause how we feel physically can be influenced by our thoughts, and what's going on in our bodies can completely change the way we think or feel about our lives.

What I've seen over and over again while working with women at all stages of the menopausal journey is that hormonal imbalances tend to be involved in almost every medical, emotional, mental, and spiritual change that women go through in midlife — whether those hormonal imbalances are "subclinical" (not shown in a test at the time the test is administered), self-diagnosed, or confirmed by a doctor.

The way imbalances tend to appear as symptoms is often related to the things in our lives we'd like to fix — like our relationships, jobs, and the personas we project out into the world; like problems that have been bothering us for years; or like stressful situations that have only recently come up. In other words, the symptoms we have often point to the very things that are bothering us.

*Exciting new initiatives in research into alternative medicine and the growth of functional and integrative medicine practices give hope that we'll be understanding this more in the coming years.*

## MY STORY — HOW I WAS ITCHING TO GET OUT

When I started my own personal journey through menopause 12 years ago, I would have told you, "I *only* want to lose weight. Don't bother me with all this psychological stuff. Don't tell me how my thinking's got to change. I don't even *want* to think about that other stuff. I *just* want a body that's 50 or 60 pounds lighter."

But even as I was concentrating on losing weight, which had side effects of getting healthy and rebalancing my hormones, my changing body demanded that I sit up and take notice, that I change my life for the better, recapture my health, rekindle the radiance of my spirit, and open myself to love. Even though I was doing the right things and moving in the right direction, new symptoms kept urging me to go even further in the right direction.

My body (and my mind and heart along with it) was talking to me, in the only language it has: symptoms and problems. It wanted me to take notice. Over and over, my body was telling me, "Something's wrong. Fix me." And, my body was doing the talking for the rest of me, as well.

It wasn't only nutrition and movement and stress that needed fixing. There were fundamental things wrong elsewhere in my life. My symptoms showed me where.

At one point during perimenopause, I got an intense case of the "itchies," right around the time I was realizing how unsatisfying my job was. At the same time, my ability to concentrate on the task at hand — the job I was supposed to be doing — disappeared. The desire to move away from what had been a rewarding business career into one centered on doing coaching around fitness, wellness, and, ultimately, menopause mastery was awakening in me. By that time, my heart had hardened (I hadn't cried, except for tearing up over sappy commercials, in more than six years). I was angry and snappish and I had mood swings. Those were my symptoms. Eventually, they led me to uncovering some of the problems that had plagued me since childhood.

I fixed all of those symptoms by shoring up my hormonal system. I did *that* by "treating" myself with great food and weight loss, by falling in love with moving my body, and by changing how stress was affecting me. I did all of the things I now work with my clients on, so they, too, can create health in their lives. But first I had to listen to the messages of the symptoms and make some other changes in my life. For me, that meant changing my job, allowing myself to open to love again by forgiving not only my ex but also others from my past, and creating practices that make my life so sweet and complete.

## WHY HORMONE REPLACEMENT THERAPY GETS IN THE WAY

I could have gone one of the other routes for dealing with my symptoms, like HRT or just toughing it out, believing that was the way things had to be. And I might have, except that I went to a new gynecologist early on. Fortunately (ultimately) for me, I was already on the path to health by then and I felt pretty good that week. He looked at my numbers, told me that things were changing (aka, I was in perimenopause), and asked if I wanted to "take something for it." I told him I was "okay for now, but I'd let him know" if things got unbearable.

I admit that, before I really got everything sorted out, there were times I was ready to say, "Just give me the magic pill!" (or the instant diet or the special skin lotion). "I'll take whatever. Just make all these symptoms go away." I wanted the hot flashes to go away. I wanted a good night's sleep. I was sick and tired of the mood swings, the anxiety, the "itchies." I wanted to not feel so old. You may be feeling pretty much the same. The main thing I felt was, "Give me back the me I used to be. I just want to be ME again!"

Although I was already doing things to get healthier and had started exercising and losing weight, I had yet to fall in love with myself, with adventure, and with the expansive possibilities available to my new, post-fifty, not-past-peri-menopause self. If I had gone on HRT, I might not have awakened to what was really going on with my body — I wouldn't have received the messages my body, mind, and heart were sending — because they wouldn't have been able to get through.

HRT dampens your body's responses to symptoms. Most women, if they're getting the right dosages of the right hormones, find relief from the worst of their symptoms. But the "cure" also dampens the message those symptoms are trying to tell you. In the 1920s and 1930s, women were institutionalized and may even been given electroshock therapy as an almost standard treatment for menopause cycle changes, and in the 1950s and 1960s, women were given tranquilizers so they wouldn't notice their symptoms. Now, HRT makes it easy to ignore the messages our bodies are sending us.

Here's why it's important to pay attention to your symptoms rather than just trying to cover them up: The more annoying and pervasive the symptom, the more you need to hear the message your inner self is trying to tell you. Even if you decide to use HRT or other interventions to relieve your symptoms, understanding if there a message in your symptoms promotes a better relationship with your body.

## HOW CAN WE HEAR THE MESSAGES?

Many people seem to believe that our thoughts and feelings are all in our heads, that it's all about the brain. But there's a broader and more insistent belief that shows up in our language. We talk about feelings in the language of parts of our bodies that aren't our brains.

The way we talk about a new love is one of the best ways to illustrate this. Take a moment to remember a time in your life when you had a new love. This doesn't have to be about a lover or a spouse. Your new love may have been for a new baby, a new pet, or an amazing project.

We feel and talk about love as if it's centered in our hearts, right? English is full of clichés like "my heart skipped a beat" and "my heart went pitter-pat." "Be still, my heart" we say when we catch sight of someone we'd love to love. And we talk of our hearts "breaking" when love goes wrong. And, it goes beyond our hearts. Love is an emotion that hits us all over our bodies. We get a feeling of "butterflies in the stomach" when we anticipate seeing him. We get "weak in the knees" when he's near. We "see only him." Those are all ways we conceive of love by noticing how it affects our bodies.

In the same way that we feel love in various parts of our bodies, other feelings and experiences find their way into our whole bodies, too. Those feelings are indicators and messages about how we *truly* feel. The key to understanding those messages is in the way our symptoms appear in our language. There are many more examples of this. Here are a few sayings that are often associated with familiar menopause symptoms:

- *"I have a gut feeling that something is wrong" (digestive issues)*

- *"I'm tied up in knots over this problem I have" (leg cramps)*

- *"My heart is broken" (heart palpitations)*

- *"I'm carrying the weight of the world" (weight gain)*

When I work with my one-on-one clients, we talk about the specific symptoms that are plaguing them. They could be hot flashes, digestive issues, weight gain, or any of a host of other symptoms. Then we look for the language cues that relate to their symptoms. As we play with the language around a symptom, my clients often feel a release as they identify the source of their symptoms in the circumstances of their life.

## NICOLE'S STORY

One of my clients, Nicole, a life coach, asked me to help her with hot flashes. Because she had already solved many of her issues around menopause through her own work in becoming a coach, we entered into a limited journey to work on this one issue.

Nicole's periods had been gone for three years and the symptoms she had experienced during perimenopause and the first year of postmenopause were gone — except for the hot flashes, which seemed unrelenting. Most days, she'd have three or four, and some of them took over her thoughts completely. When a hot flash came while she was on a client call on Skype, she'd be embarrassed by the flush of heat to her face and sometimes lose her focus.

In our first session, Nicole and I talked about her experience of menopause and why she thought she was still experiencing hot flashes. She talked about some of the steps she'd taken to eliminate the hot flashes. Because she was reluctant to take drugs and had heard about the potential risks of HRT, she wanted a natural alternative, so she'd tried eliminating the more common triggers for hot flashes from her diet (alcohol, caffeine, and spicy foods). She'd also tried other nutritional interventions, like eliminating red meat and adding soy (this is not always effective). None of those things seemed to reduce the frequency or intensity of her flashes.

Nicole had hoped that I would recommend some herbs or reassure her that the answer was to take HRT, so she was surprised when I asked her to listen to a few common phrases and see whether any of them rang true for her. Feeling "hot under the collar," an indicator of anger and rage, didn't ring true for her. We talked about embarrassment and feeling "red-faced and flustered," but, again, that didn't feel right for her. The one that seems to cause my own hot flashes — "having an excess of energy" — didn't strike a chord with Nicole, either.

It wasn't until we started talking about exercise and how it relates to hot flashes by helping to reduce them that Nicole told me she hated exercising. I asked why, and she told me she hated getting all sweaty. "After all, nobody likes to sweat," she said. There it was! We played around with phrases about sweating and the one that really rang true for her was, "Don't let them see you sweat." Starting her coaching business had been a stretch for her, and she wanted to appear experienced and in control.

We made a few adjustments in Nicole's diet, got her started on a movement program she loved (at an air-conditioned gym!), and I helped her find an accountability partner who would provide support and encouragement when Nicole's trepidation began to overwhelm her. The last time we spoke, her hot flashes had subsided and she'd learned to appreciate that the remaining hot flashes let her know when she was moving into uncomfortable territory in her business.

## LISTENING TO YOUR SYMPTOMS, DISCOVERING YOUR STORIES

Are you interested in getting to the bottom of your symptoms? Here's a journaling exercise I use with my clients to help them dig into what's going on. Sometimes I'll have them start with journaling for a couple of weeks to determine the patterns of their symptoms, and then we'll talk about the answers to the questions below in a one-on-one session. For other clients (like Nicole), the symptoms and the patterns are more easily accessible because they're already almost conscious about them, and we work through the symptom's messages and the questions below in one session.

So, grab your journal. Think about the symptoms that are bothering you and answer the following questions about each of them:

- **What is the symptom?** Give it a full description. Where in your body do you feel it? Do you see it as a symptom of your body, mind, heart, and/or spirit?

- **How do you rate the level of your annoyance with this symptom?** Use whatever rating scale you want, but include whether it's always, sometimes, or rarely annoying.

- **When did you first notice this symptom?** Is it something you noticed right away or through an awareness that grew on you? Is this symptom constant or intermittent? Can you tell if there's a pattern related to its appearance?

At this point, you'll want to decide whether to take some time journaling about this symptom for a few days or longer, in order to gather more information about how it appears in your life. If the symptom is fairly constant, you may not need to journal about it; you may already have all the information you need. If the symptom is intermittent and recurs with a pattern, you may need to journal through the whole pattern. Many symptoms have patterns that revolve around the menstrual cycle, so you may need to journal as long as an entire cycle, or even more than one.

Here are more questions to consider to help you notice whether you experience a specific symptom in a day:

- **Did I experience the symptom today?** If you did, was there a triggering event? What was happening just prior to the appearance of this symptom? If you didn't experience this symptom today, was there anything that you noticed that might be related to its absence?

- **Did I eat anything that might have triggered or suppressed this symptom?** Some of the foods or beverages to consider that might be having an effect are sugared or artificially sweetened soft drinks, alcohol, sugar, wheat, dairy, red meat, and caffeine. A specific type of alcohol or other drink or food may be a trigger.

- **What was my general mood today?** Did you feel good or bad today? How were you feeling before this symptom appeared?

Once you have information from answering the above sets of questions, it's time to figure out what's going on!

Set aside some quiet time where you won't be disturbed (if you can't find a quiet hour, that's pretty telling, isn't it?). Sit with your journal and review your findings in the following ways.

- **Describe the symptom as graphically as you can.** Use words that are as specific as possible. This is going to help out as you look for "sayings" that might give you clues about what's going on.

- **Riff on your symptom.** Think about and jot down anything that seems related to this symptom — common sayings, related feelings, synonyms for your descriptive words, other times in your life when you felt this way, how this symptom makes you feel, other things that cause you to feel this same way. Write it all down. Don't try to be neat, just scribble it all down as fast as it comes. Don't edit, and include things even if they don't feel quite right.

- **Now edit what you wrote.** What does feel right? What doesn't quite explain this symptom for you? Watch for anything you dismiss too quickly. Sometimes this indicates a situation you're avoiding noticing. Usually, as you edit what you jotted in the last step, you'll see something that either screams yes or that screams no so loudly you're pretty sure you're avoiding it. Circle anything that stands out for you.

- **Play with the words, phrases, and sayings that stand out.** Try to understand how these apply to your life. I will warn you that sometimes a symptom is just a symptom and doesn't "mean" anything. Also, sometimes a symptom does have a message about your life, but you might not find it right away. That's okay. If no meaning for this symptom comes up, skip the next step.

- **Plan an approach to reducing the impact of the underlying situation on your life.** This might include setting boundaries around an annoying situation, practicing in order to make something you need to do easier, or using stress-reduction techniques about something that can't be changed.

- **Plan an approach for reducing the effects of the symptom.** Understanding the reason a symptom may be showing up, and even fixing the problem it stems from, might not make the symptom go away. For example, when I learned that my symptom of regaining weight felt consistent with feeling that I was "carrying the weight of the world on my back," that didn't make the weight go away overnight. I still had to, and continue to have to, do the work to lose it.

I've created a free "mini-course" called Reveal the Roadblock for you to help you work with this technique. If you'll set aside just a couple hours, I will help you examine one symptom and the message it has for you. Beginning with a guided meditation, you can detach from the sensation of annoyance, while examining the symptom from a place of compassion and understanding. Then, I'll guide you through the rest of the process and help you discover the messages your symptoms have for you. You can get the course at www.menopause.guru/rtr.

Once you listen to the messages of your body, heart, and mind, you'll find yourself opening up to the idea that maybe it *is* possible to find yourself again. Even during menopause.

# CHAPTER 9

# EVE'S GIFT

When I first started learning about the process of menopause, I was, to be honest, horrified by the sheer number and diversity of symptoms I might experience. The idea of all those things happening to me at once was scary, and I admit that I felt a fair amount of panic.

Maybe you're like I was. You're looking at this journey and thinking you'd rather not board that train. Or, if you're already on board, maybe you're looking for the next station so you can disembark. The problem is that not taking the journey isn't really an option.

Here's the thing: If you're looking at menopause through the eyes of fear, it can seem pretty scary. You may be wanting to surrender to that fear and refuse to deal with the changes. You may be wanting to fight back, to try to hang onto the you that you were, refusing to give in to the changes that are changing you. But no amount of insisting on being the same you that you've been is going to keep menopause from happening.

## CHANGE HAPPENS

No matter how hard you fight it, change is going to happen. The truth is that change is happening to us all the time. You know that old saw (*really* old — Heraclitus, ca. 500 BCE, was the author of this quote), "You can't step into the same river twice, for other rivers are ever flowing on to you." The *essence* of life is change.

As the world changes around you, just as it always has, you may be hoping to remain the way you are now or get back to the version of yourself that knew how to cope better. You want to be resilient enough (again) to roll with the punches and take care of everything you feel responsible for. You just want to be yourself again, right?

There's another way to look at it. Navigating well through menopause takes more than the steps we've already talked about, and there's a better way than muddling through and trying to get back to the old you.

When I took a personal vow to let my divorce become the best thing that ever happened to me, I did something more than accept the changes happening to me, even though I didn't realize it at the time. I *embraced* the changes. I opened myself up to the experiences and the potential of the (many) years left to me. I became enthusiastic about my life beyond the years I'd spent being a wife, a career woman, and a mother.

That wasn't a conscious decision about the best way to get to happiness. I really *didn't* think I had a choice. My ex was most definitely an ex. Even if I'd wanted to reconcile, when my ex closes a door behind him, he slams it and triple locks it. That relationship was gone. My house was gone. I was on to a new job. Change had happened. So I had to change *myself* to fit into the new world I was already in.

Back there was the old me, the one who knew all the wonders and beauties of being a wife and a mother, someone designed to be the center of the family, to hold together its diverse members and nourish them. I was also a businesswoman, a consultant working in the computer industry. But, as rewarding as that was, it had also been all-consuming.

This new me? I'm still everything I was, but I'm also more. Today, I'm everything I choose to be.

## HOW DID WE GET HERE?

The big changes in our reproductive systems mark big changes in who we are in the world. Puberty marks the change between "little girl" and "adulthood." Perhaps someone told you "Now you're a woman" when you had your first period. At that time, your hormones, especially estrogen, pushed you to concentrate on being a nurturer. Estrogen triggers us to focus on babies and boys, and we become more willing to be the peacemaker and the home-creator.

If you bore children, the hormones of pregnancy marked your transition to motherhood. Estrogen and progesterone flooded your system, preparing you for childbirth. As you held your child for the first time, oxytocin reinforced your bond with your child.

As our reproductive systems wind down, the influence of estrogen recedes. The need to be the nurturer, homemaker, and people-pleaser starts to subside. Those roles, which we've held for so long (even when we've also had careers and community positions), start to move out of the center of existence, and the child we once were starts to re-emerge.

## EVE'S GIFT

What I've learned in the years following my divorce and during my passage through menopause — what I continue to learn — is that we women have been given a magnificent gift in menopause. This is Eve's gift. Whether you believe in a literal Eve or not, evolution has gifted us with a magnificent "change of life." As we leave childbearing behind, we also leave behind the effects of estrogen on our brains.

Because we change so completely as our hormones change during menopause, and because that affects every part of our being, we have an opportunity to reinvent ourselves, to wrap every possibility, every dream, every hope and desire, and every achievement that's ever been ours into a new, more authentic self.

Don't get me wrong. We still love our children. We still value our marriages, homes, and careers. We'd still walk through fire if it would help our kids. But we're starting to recognize that there's more here, more to us, than just our family. We're really somebody, too. We have ideas and ambitions, and there are perhaps possibilities we've been attracted to but never fully explored. Most importantly, we have the same right and responsibility as everyone else to shine our light in the world.

In the previous chapter, I talked about how our symptoms talk to us, how sometimes they're telling us about relationships that aren't serving us or that it's time to do something else, something new. Our symptoms may be telling us we have a message for the world that we aren't yet voicing. Our symptoms speak of changes we need to make — not because the person we were was wrong, but because it's time to be even more deeply and genuinely ourselves.

I recently spoke with a woman at a workshop who was nearing retirement. She held a prominent position at a local university, where she was responsible for much of the physical plant. I asked her, "What have you done that you're most proud of?" This lovely lady, who'd done so much in her own right, told me, "My grandbaby."

If you give me half a second, I'll tell you how excited I am to be welcoming my first grandbaby into the world this fall. Yes, I'm proud of my son, his wife, and their little boy. If I asked you what you've done that you're most proud of, your first reaction might be to tell me about the accomplishments of your children, your grandchildren, or even your husband. The pride you take in what others who are close to you do or who they are is justifiable pride in their accomplishments. Yes, you've contributed, but, ultimately, they are responsible for the accomplishments of their own lives.

Of course, those aren't your only accomplishments. It's time to recognize that you have gifts of your own to share with the world. For many, if not most of us, the achievements of our childbearing years are locked in with the achievements of our families — our children and our spouses. And yet... and yet, we're so much more.

In this chapter, I'll give you tools to help you awaken your new self, incorporate your old self, bond with the person you're becoming, and embrace this awesome new creation — *you*!

## REKINDLING THE FLAME OF YOUR DREAMS

The germ of who you can be is hidden inside the you that you are today and the you that you were as a child. But it may be that you've forgotten the passions you had back then. When you were so busy raising your children and making a living and being a responsible adult, the things you felt passionate about may not have seemed as important. They might even have seemed immature or selfish.

It's time to take out those old dreams again, to feel the zest for something that's uniquely yours. It's time to rekindle the flame (is that what the hot flashes are telling you?) inside you and for you!

Unfortunately, sometimes we've moved so far from our true desires that we've forgotten they're in there. And our desires may have changed over the years. Perhaps we've combined them with new desires in marvelous ways, and we haven't quite seen that yet. When we go on this journey of menopause, it's almost magic how all the pieces start to fit together.

Begin with looking back in time to find and recapture the child and the girl and the young woman you were, examining the things that made their heart, your heart, sing. Listen to the siren song that's calling you now. Take a look — not only in your mind's eye, but also in reality — at the vistas you'd like to travel. Feel the excitement you felt then and the excitement you dream of feeling.

## YOUR INNER CHILD'S VISION BOARD

A vision board is a technique that can help you focus on the things you'd like to be, do, and have in your life, by gathering images and words from magazines and other sources and gluing them to a surface to create a collage that speaks to you. If your inner child hasn't had a chance to come out and play in a while, creating a vision board is a great way to connect with her. It can keep you from missing the dreams you most want to fulfill.

I'd like to add a word about forgiveness here. Often when I work with clients in this process, negative memories from childhood arise, even for women who had exceedingly happy childhoods. That happened to me as I created a vision board for my inner child. Sometimes, a forgiveness practice is necessary to facilitate letting go and moving into the world that's opening up to you now.

I know that forgiving is something that we hear a lot about. Almost every spiritual practice or religious framework recommends it. But, for me, it was always a whole lot harder than just saying, "I forgive you." How do you actually *do* it? Recently, I discovered a process that actually works — it's not a spiritual thesis about why to forgive; it's an actual practical, step-by-step process that allows you to change the emotions around the hurt. You can download a guide to this process at www.menopause.guru/forgive/.

When I work with my clients to create their inner child vision board, we start with a few minutes of quiet remembering, reaching back to a time when daydreaming was easy and fun and the possibility of achieving dreams seemed endless. As you do this, I recommend using a photo of yourself as you were then, to help you center on the perspective of this little girl. It works best if you can find a picture of yourself as you were then, but it also works to find a stock image of a girl who could be your inner child (or you can use this one: www.menopause.guru/child) to trigger your imagination.

With a journal or blank paper close at hand, start with looking at the picture of yourself or of a young girl that you've selected. Allow your thoughts to wander back to her time. If you weren't given much opportunity for doing this type of daydreaming as a child, see if you can idealize it — imagine what it would have been like to daydream when you were a girl. Connect with that little girl of limitless possibilities. Give over control of all of your memories to your inner child, no matter when those memories happened in your life. Memories from any age up to now are fair game.

As quickly as you can, capture the memories, writing down things you've done or been or had that really made your inner child happy. Write quickly, just a word or two to capture the memory. Allow yourself to linger on things that felt particularly important, to see if there are more aspects of that happiness that you can capture. Remember that the memories may be from any time in your life.

I'll give you an example of how this works. My inner child is about seven years old. When I did this exercise and let go and remembered the things that make her happy, some of the things on my list (and the age I was) were: horses (always), dogs (12), camping (14), reading (always), running through the woods (11), writing (12), skiing (24), acting (15), and quilting (35). And, yes, there were a lot more things than those on my list!

The next step is to capture and list the things you've wanted to try, but have never had the chance to. It doesn't matter why you haven't done them. If you always wanted to swim with dolphins, but never got out of Nebraska, or were told by your piano teacher you'd never be a concert pianist, or just thought it would be fun to be a firefighter — that's okay! Now is the time to put it on your list anyway, because you can, and because your dreams are important and full of clues.

Stay with asking your inner child these questions: What would she like to try? What would she like to be? What would make her happy? Some of the things that come up may trigger a need for forgiveness, especially if they were things you did have for a while but then were taken from you. See what comes up for you here around this. Remember the horse that was on my list? Nope, I never had one of my own. I still don't. There are a lot of reasons for this, but "horse" remains on my list (and on my vision board!).

Now that you have a list of combined experiences and wishes, look for trends and things that have come back into your life in new and surprising ways. It's amazing how things show up. Dance shows up on my list. Here's a story about dance in my life. When I was in about third grade, I went to a day camp where we got to try lots of different stuff (everything from archery to building clay pots). For one of the sessions, I chose to try ballet. I was fascinated by dance and thought I'd be a natural. I wasn't. My natural athletic ineptitude shone through. That was a different era, and "Madame," the very proper French ballet teacher, told me quite bluntly that I should not bother trying to continue with lessons. I was devastated and I didn't dance much for the next 50 years. Even when I became a fitness professional, I refused to even try to teach any of the myriad of dance-based exercise programs. I once tripped up a whole row in a demonstration Zumba class!

I avoided dance until I ran into a type of fitness class called Nia. Nia is an expressive dance workout with roots in many dance and movement styles. My Nia teacher encouraged me to express myself in movement, to just enjoy what my body felt like doing. She taught me to hear the beat that had always eluded me, and my inner child sang, because *this* was the dance I'd been looking for all these years! My Nia teacher said to me, "I'm offering teacher training and you would be perfect to teach this." So, yes, I teach Nia now!

Dance is absolutely on my inner child vision board.

Mark up the lists you made from remembering what your passions have been and what you wish you could do. Circle the important stuff. Cross off stuff that doesn't even make any sense any more. Connect the dots where you see patterns and notice how things fit together now. Add other things you think of as you play with your list.

Now it's time to create your vision board, using your marked-up list as a guide. Get a big piece of poster board, foam-core board, or even one of those tri-fold science project boards. Grab a bunch of magazines, markers, glitter pens, yarn, and anything else you'd like to use to create your board. You'll also need scissors and some type of glue, like glue sticks or spray glue, to stick it all together.

You might want to put your picture of your inner child on the board. Maybe in the center, or in a corner. Maybe with thought bubbles coming out of her/your head. Do whatever works for you.

Look through magazines for pictures and words that illustrate the things on your list, especially ones that spark the deepest feelings of passion and joy when you imagine doing, being, and having it.

As you look through magazines, you may find pictures that trigger other thoughts and desires. Some may be true to your inner child, but beware of being distracted by shiny things — things that attract you, but aren't really you. Maybe you get excited about a picture that's a possibility, but is really only a bauble — something you like, but isn't really a part of your deep vision. For example, I might see a picture of a diamond ring and think, "Wow, that's really pretty. I want that." But, I really don't. Not in a Big Vision sort of way. Or maybe I see a photo of someone climbing Mt. Everest and wonder if I could do that. Wondering is fine, but unless I would really like to do it and imagining doing it gives me a deep, happy feeling, it doesn't belong on this vision board.

Be sure the things on your vision board are true to your inner child's sense of joy and passion. Then let your board help you to guide your actions to bring these desires into or back into your life.

## DISPEL THE FEAR OF LIVING YOUR DREAMS

The biggest reason we fight the change of menopause is fear. We fear we'll lose the life we have and we're not sure there's anything more for us out there once we've changed our identity from "wife and mother" to whatever's next.

But if we go ahead and *choose* what's next, and choose to take action to make what we want to happen actually happen, then this next portion of our lives can be the best part yet, because we take everything we were and add in everything we want to be. We keep the best from before, and we accept the changes we're going through, so that we become the best we've ever been.

And that is Eve's gift to us!

# CHAPTER 10

# WHO'S ON YOUR TEAM?

There are teams all around us, from sports teams to project teams on the job. We see businesses advertising their customer service teams. Your kids have probably been on teams most of their lives, and you may have used the "family as team" concept when you explained why they needed to clean up their rooms or why that pony they wanted wasn't in the family budget or wouldn't fit in your New York City apartment.

We teach our kids teamwork. It makes things easier and more fun. It makes less work for any one person when everyone contributes what they have and what they know. In the end, you get lots better results, for everybody.

And yet, when it comes to our own lives, we somehow think we have to do it all ourselves. We have to be our sole source of support — the strong, silent type. John Wayne had nothing on most women, huh? We'll cry at the drop of a hat over a TV commercial, but you'll never know about *our* suffering.

Maybe you've long been the super competent one. If you didn't already know how to do it, you looked it up and got busy figuring it out. You grabbed a cookbook or a manual and read the instructions. What you produced may not have come out looking exactly like the picture, but sometimes it was even better!

Except now the changes you're going through have you befuddled. We don't have a manual personal enough to cover the things that are happening to our particular bodies as we go through menopause. But our hearts are crying out for care — care from ourselves and care from those who are important to us. We feel the urge to connect to our own spirits in deeper ways, but maybe don't know how.

The truth is, going it alone, doing it all by ourselves isn't going to cut it anymore.


## WE NEED A TEAM

An article on weight loss I read recently reported a finding that the researchers hadn't expected. They'd listed every habit, practice, or trick they knew that was used to lose weight and maintain the loss (over 160 different items!). Then they asked weight-loss coaches to rate the methods their clients used successfully.

The number one answer wasn't even on the list!

There were a lot of good methods for achieving and maintaining weight loss, but, overwhelmingly, the most important element was "support." Not, as you might expect, the support of close family and friends, but the support of people outside that close circle. Meaningful support, support that really made a difference, came from strangers (who often became friends in the process) and coaches who provided accountability, support, and knowledge during the process of losing weight.

The answer may have surprised the researchers, but it didn't surprise the weight-loss coaches. It doesn't surprise me either. I learned the power of support as I went through my own menopausal and weight-loss journey. And the support I found continues to help me today.

Over the past ten years, I've assembled my own support team. It's a strange kind of team. Not everybody who's on the team knows they're on it. Most of them don't know it's a menopause support team and, in truth, they support me in all kinds of ventures, not just the menopause adventure. The people on my team don't all know each other, and I've never even met a good chunk of them. Several people on my team have no idea who I am.

My team is ever-expanding and made up of people from all over the world. Over the years, I've met many of them in person. I may never meet some of them, and I just might "fire" a few here and there. Even so, it's the best team in the world for me!

## MY TEAM

I have a few medical people on my team, like my primary care doctor, my gynecologist from where I lived before my divorce, my current nurse practitioner, and a great chiropractor. Not all doctors make good team members. Some of the doctors I've seen during this time of going through menopause didn't make it onto my team. Some of them had no idea what menopause's changes meant. Others thought dispensing a pill was the only answer for dealing with my symptoms. My team only includes the doctors and medical professionals who are good for me.

Also on my team are some great wellness helpers: several good massage therapists (who've helped me learn to enjoy being touched again), a few "mean" personal trainers, and a couple of great running coaches. Eventually, I added a therapist to my team and 2 fabulous life coaches, in addition to several amazing workshop presenters and motivational speakers.

A few amazing friends — new and old friends — who've done so much to help me (including driving my two cats to Alabama from New Hampshire!) are members of my team. Some friends have stayed in my life and some aren't around anymore, but I've been blessed by all the friends on my team.

I belong to a world-class (and world-wide) peer support network. These are women I didn't discover until I was trying to lose weight and cope with divorce and menopause and a new job, all at the same time. They gave generously of themselves when I was still a stranger, and asked nothing in return except that I do the same.

And, yes, books are on my team, as is the Internet, where I gain support from authors, especially Dr. Christiane Northrup, the late Dr. John Lee, and Dr. Louann Brizendine. I count them as part of my support team.

## NOT MY TEAM

Let's talk about people who don't belong on my team, and why. My ex-husband, for example, was never on my team. Our relationship was crumbling long before I went into perimenopause and my reactions to it (along with some outside pressures) finished us off. When I looked to him for accountability, I put an extra strain on our relationship because *I* didn't really want to be accountable. When he called me out on something, it just made me mad. And when I needed his support, he didn't understand what I was going through.

A couple of "false friends" and a few relatives aren't on my team. Not everyone in your life wants what is best for you. For example, my mom wasn't on my support team. If she were someone different, I would have loved her support. But not all moms (or aunts, older sisters, cousins, etc.) understand that your experience of menopause can be different from theirs. My mom's "pull yourself up by your bootstraps and soldier on, soldier!" attitude didn't fit with my need to *understand* what's happening.

My son fits into this category, too. (He's my only child.) He's had his own stuff going on during these years when I've been going through menopause. He's been finishing college, dealing with his parents' divorce, establishing a career, getting married. His support and love have been absolutely amazing and essential, but, for the most part, I can't lean on him, because he's got his own life and this is *not* an issue for which you can ask your child's support, especially your boy child.

My current husband is sweet, lovable, and the best friend I've ever had. He supports me in a thousand ways every day. He even listens as I process all this stuff and work to understand it. But he's on a different team, the same team my mom, son, dad, cats, and dog were and are on. This is not the team that holds me accountable or listens to my weirder rants, or helps me figure out exactly what my next step is. My husband is on the unconditional love team — another great team to have, by the way!

## WHO DO YOU NEED ON YOUR TEAM?

Of course, I can't tell you who the best people are to fill the slots on your menopause support team, but I *can* suggest some slots you might want to consider filling:

Friends who "get it." Often, our friends are a great first line of defense, especially women friends who are around the same age. They can help answer questions like, "Did this happen to you?" and "Is this normal?" and "Do you know a good fix for this?" and "What do you do about it?" They don't always know the answer, but good friends will support you, anyway.

They can also provide a listening ear for the ever-popular need to "*Please* let me rant about my husband (kids, friends, boss, co-workers)!"

Yes, you need friends who understand you. Absolutely. They're your cheerleaders and your encouragers. They love you. And you love them back. (And if they don't love you, maybe it's time for new ones!)

Remember what Groucho Marx said: "When you're in jail, a good friend will be trying to bail you out. A best friend will be in the cell next to you saying, 'Damn, that was fun.'" Yep, you absolutely need to have fun with your friends. But when you want to stay out of trouble, a best friend may not be as helpful as a friend who can bail you out. Ask yourself if your friends are helping or hurting. Who are the friends you want on your menopause support team?

**Peer support groups.** Support groups around any cause or issue or problem are everywhere these days. You can find them on social media or at local community centers or at churches. If you're trying to change something, they can make fabulous teammates.

Many of the best support group members have a lot of experience dealing with the things you're going through, and they're willing to share and offer support and help and suggest alternatives.

**Experts.** I've got to say that great doctors and nurse practitioners will make your menopausal journey so much easier. They'll understand your personal approach to your body and your health. They'll calm your fears and provide simple alternatives to feeling trapped in illness or various kinds of disability. They're the ones who can recognize when something might be going way off track and require intervention.

What other experts do you want on your team? A good massage therapist, a great hair stylist, a tough personal trainer? Maybe a skin-care expert? These kinds of people can help you look and feel great as you make changes. They pamper you and help you concentrate on yourself and feeling good in your body.

**Great books by great authors.** Information is now more available than ever. My Kindle is loaded with great advice on topics from dog training to organizing my house and my time (a never-ending battle, I'm afraid) to how to read hormone tests. When I need information about what's happening to me, in any area of my life, I often turn to books.

## SUPPORT TEAM PITFALLS

I read and even comment in a lot of online support groups about menopause and perimenopause. Many of these groups are named things like Menopause Misery, Perimenopause Hell, and Menopause Sucks. Many of them provide a useful service to the women who hang out in them. They provide information (although not necessarily expertise, because the information often hasn't been checked for accuracy), commiseration, and reassurance, especially during health crises.

But they also reinforce the idea that menopause is miserable. Many of the women in these groups are unhappy with their experience but don't see a way out. This type of group results from a combination of things. Partly, they get mired in the negativity and new women joining the group take on the group's perspective and repeat old problems. Women who solve the problems for themselves leave the group. And experts aren't really a part of that network, so the information that appears in them isn't necessarily reliable.

The peer pressure in these groups keeps up the myth that menopause is a negative experience. This is what one group member said her reaction was when a friend asked her what perimenopause is: "I walked away. I couldn't be the one to give her the news of the absolute hell she was getting ready to endure."

## WHAT'S THE SUPPORT GROUP SOLUTION?

Every great team needs someone taking a look at the big picture and helping to direct the action — someone who holds you accountable for the actions you've said you'll take; someone who helps you let go of your stories and excuses; someone who helps you hold on to the vision of your possibilities and dreams.

Recently, a friend posted this on her Facebook feed: "Making changes that last *requires* deep digging, honesty with self, and accountability to make the new choices a habit. This is where a guide, a coach, a mentor comes in. Finding someone you trust, who *hears* you, and who you feel safe with, is critical to your success." (Jennifer Nearents)

Jennifer was talking about her own journey, but she could easily be talking about mine. I've been blessed with having great coaches in any number of areas in my life (diet and fitness, business, and personal growth, to name just a few).

The kind of coaching I'm talking about is like the coaches of old-school football teams, long before the days of earphones in the quarterbacks' helmets, before the coach sent in every play from the bench. All week long, those coaches helped the players understand the problems they'd face, helped them develop their talents and perfect their skills, so that they could make decisions on their own during the game. Then, when the game started, the coach would help when things went wrong, suggest a strategy change during a time-out, or send in a team member to help. But, ultimately, the players on the field had to make their own decisions.

A great coach helps you see your possibilities, go beyond what you see as your limitations, and actually achieve your goals. A great coach helps you focus on your vision and keeps you moving toward it, helping you correct your course when you get off track.

## THE FOUR PILLARS REVISITED

Thriving during menopause and beyond takes more than just thinking and believing. It takes more than prescriptions for HRT or anti-depressants. It even takes more than understanding what's happened to create the *dis-ease* in your life that's showing up as symptoms. It takes action to build support for yourself as a whole woman. We've been busy taking care of everyone else, and sometimes it can seem like that's been our whole life, but now it's time to take care of ourselves more. I'll remind you of the four pillars that can help you do that.

We've talked about the nutrition pillar — how selecting the right foods to support you and matching them to your hormonal needs right now boosts your health and helps you feel great. Sometimes that means putting in effort to change the way you eat and to figure out what great foods to choose for your new, great body. Supporting yourself might even mean losing weight. It's only a myth that losing weight and keeping it off is impossible once you start menopausal changes. You really can be your best self ever!

Then there's the pillar of movement — selecting movement that delights your body and that you love to do, taking time to have fun and experience adventures, stepping beyond what you do normally, and being active. You may need to change how you move your body to absolutely support the person you're becoming.

The third pillar is about relaxing and figuring out how stress can be managed. Understanding where your stressors come from and changing them can help, but so many of the stressors may seem out of your control. What *is* in your control is how you respond to them. By controlling your reaction to the things life sends your way, you open up the ability to create a new outcome — one with a positive and lasting impact.

Finally, the fourth pillar is getting the support you need. Don't go it alone! There is help out there for you. Connecting with your friends, your peers, the experts, and getting the help of a great coach make going through these challenging changes much easier. You're much more likely to wind up with the results you want: a you that's everything you were and more — everything you'd like to be!

# CHAPTER 11

# YOU 2.0

I suspect you started reading this book because you wanted to go back to being the person you were before menopause, perimenopause, or postmenopause came along. But I wrote this book because I want you to understand the changes going on in your body, so that you can decide who you want to be for the rest of your life. Because it's up to you. It's your choice. And it's about so much more than going back to who you were.

In recent generations, there have been two common paths through menopause: traditional medical treatments and toughing it out.

For the past century, women have gone to their doctors with their menopause symptoms and said, "Fix me." This is the interaction model we've adopted with our medical professionals in general, whether what's bothering us is the flu, a broken arm, or a chronic illness. So our doctors attempt to "fix" us. They prescribe hormones or antidepressants or, in some cases, even surgery to remove the offensive parts.

Medical treatments may take the edge off your symptoms. Sometimes, your symptoms can disappear altogether through medical treatment. You can even get back to feeling like yourself again. But HRT, psychotropic drugs, and surgery generally don't get you to glowing health, to feeling truly terrific about yourself, or to fulfilling the dreams of your heart. And some of those medical treatments include rather scary side effects.

Another common option for women going through menopause is to "tough it out." This was the option used when the whole family had the flu and *someone* had to make the chicken soup and deliver the fluids and take the temperatures and wash the dishes and feed the dog, even though they were sick, too. About 100 percent of the time, that was mom, right? We assume we know how to keep going, no matter what. Just power through and ignore the symptoms until they go away.

The problem with that way of dealing with menopause is that our symptoms arise from a place deeper than germs that give us the flu. So often, our symptoms really are our souls screaming at us to take notice, to take time for ourselves, to fill up the well we've depleted in all our years of caring for everyone else. When we continue to ignore them, they only keep screaming louder.

I offer you a different path than medical treatments or toughing it out. It's the path of self-care and reconnecting with the parts of yourself that may have been lost while you were being everything to everyone in your life. This is the path of using nutrition and movement and stress management to balance your hormones and support your health. This is about looking into finding your comfortable weight. It's certainly about increasing your ability to perform everyday tasks by relying on the four pillars (nutrition or diet, movement, stress management, and support) to continue to deliver wonderful, positive side effects that keep multiplying.

This is the path of self-love and self-esteem, of caring about yourself enough to take care of yourself, of knowing and believing you are worth your investment in yourself.

This is the path of recapturing all the dreams of your life and tuning in to which ones you still want to make come true, and then making them come true, in whatever way makes sense to you now. This is the path to You 2.0, the you that encompasses all you've been up until now and every possibility you're open to for the rest of your life.

The you that you've been up until now is a fascinating and fabulous woman. There's no denying that! (I maintain this as truth, even if you just snorted when you read that, even if you aren't ready to give yourself that credit yet.) You've done amazing things. Some of them in your own right, but I'll bet a whole lot more were about helping others to be their best selves — your kids, your spouse, your community, your co-workers. They've all benefited from you!

Maybe, just maybe, it's time for someone to take care of you. That someone is *you*. And who could be better for that job, because you really *do* know best what you need. A doctor will want you to take a test — a blood test or an EKG or some other test. That may help with a piece of the solution, but wouldn't you rather give yourself a test, by tuning in to your own inner voice and telling yourself the answers you most need to hear? You *know* the answers. You only need to uncover them.

Over the past few chapters, I've shared with you some of the most important answers I've found in my journey through menopause to health and happiness. These are the "secrets" (yeah, as you saw, they aren't really secrets) I use to help my Menopause Mastery clients recapture themselves and go beyond to their best selves ever.

When I started my Menopause Mastery coaching program, I went searching for a wonderful, uplifting synonym for menopause that would resonate with and encourage the women I work with. I read books, searched the Internet, delved into dictionaries and thesauruses (thesauri?), asked my older women friends, and read dozens of book descriptions on Amazon. I even searched through scholarly texts on myth and folktales to see how they described post-menopausal women. I have to say that the results were discouraging! In fact, alternate terms for "menopause" were so sparse and had such negative connotations that I wouldn't want to use them.

So, I've created my own term: "Midlife Nirvana." I don't use the word "nirvana" in any religious sense. But that word does describe the type of peace, happiness, and deep-seated joy I think we're searching for during this time in our lives. I define "Midlife Nirvana" as a state of being "at peace with your past, engaged in your present, and excited about your future."

When we're in the state of Midlife Nirvana, we're at peace with our past, because we realize that our path was exactly the right path to bring us to where we are today. We know there are things left undone in our lives, but we also know that there's still time. We know we can resurrect our old dreams, cherish them for what they bring to us today, and fulfill them.

In Midlife Nirvana, we're engaged in our present. We practice the self-care needed in order to be healthy and vibrant, whether we're already there or not. We're balanced in our approach to our bodies, minds, hearts, and spirits, so that, as changes happen and symptoms appear, we recognize them for what they are — messages to take care of ourselves, to notice what we need right now, and to take steps to meet those needs, whether that means setting boundaries in a relationship or finding a better face cream.

In Midlife Nirvana, we're excited about our future. We know that now is our time to shine and that we have the resources and capabilities to be amazing in our own right while still being a vibrant part of the lives of those we care about. We know that our future is just as exciting and fulfilling as our today, because we're taking action to create our future.

I invite you to embark on your own quest for Midlife Nirvana. Take control of your menopausal journey by making self-care (taking the nutrition, movement, and stress-management steps I've talked about in this book) a priority. Take the next step to clarify what you'd most love to do with the rest of your life, because it's *your* life to live!

It's your choice. You can continue trying to tough it out. You can go to a doctor and get pills that may or may not be effective or safe. Or you can use the knowledge and tools in this book to take control of your own menopausal journey. You can make a difference in your own life, help your body do what it's designed to do, and open yourself to the possibilities of the rest of your life.

If you make the choice to support your body, listen to your symptoms, and embrace this time of your life with enthusiasm, I guarantee you'll fall in love with You 2.0!

# ACKNOWLEDGMENTS

I am profoundly grateful to the members of my support team, for all their assistance, encouragement, and belief in the work I do and the dreams I seek to fulfill.

From the very start, I found accountability, support, and friendship with the members and staff of the pre-2010 eDiets crew. I'd especially like to thank Cathy Cox and Raphael Calzadilla for their ever-willingness to answer questions and provide new goals to challenge me. My peer mentor groups, especially The Mavens, The Wonder Women, and The Fitness Fanatics, were and, in many cases, are terrific friends and motivators.

Without the assistance, in book form, of some amazing authors, my journey would have been far more rugged. I would like to thank Dr. Christiane Northrup, Dr. Louann Brizendine, and Dr. John Lee for the knowledge and awareness they have so graciously spread in the world. Their work has formed the basis of my understanding and my health and underlies the totality of this book.

I've been the beneficiary of some amazing coaching — in particular, from Amira Alvarez, Elaine Bailey, and Nyali Muir — all of whom do amazing work in the world.

Anyone who hopes to make a difference in the world could do no better than to harness the power of the staff and founder of The Difference Press. Without the help of Angela Lauria, Grace Kerina, and the others there, you would be reading a very different and much less useful book (if I even finished it in the first place!).

My gratitude goes out to Kate Finlayson, who opened the world of dance to me and taught me that there are many paths to passion!

There's no way this book could have been written without any of the members of my unconditional-love support team: Jesse, Jamie, Kate, and Miles. I love each of them in the way I know they love me — unconditionally and forever.

Lastly, I would like to thank Rich, for making the decision I could have never made, but which started me on the journey that led me here.

# ABOUT THE AUTHOR

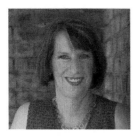

Jeanne Andrus is bursting with a passion for helping women come through their menopausal journey with renewed health and an excitement for the life they may have thought was gone forever.

After years of neglecting herself while pursuing motherhood and a corporate career, Jeanne committed to health and self-fulfillment at the age of 48, in the wake of a divorce. Her newfound love for fitness and health helped her lose 80 pounds, renew her passion for outdoor adventure, and create the life of her dreams.

That dream included creating a business as a personal trainer and health coach (certified by the American Council on Exercise). Coaching women around fitness and weight loss led Jeanne to realize how pervasive women's struggles around the changes of perimenopause and menopause are, and led her to create a holistic coaching approach to midlife that she calls Menopause Mastery Coaching.

When Jeanne's not coaching her clients, who live all over the world, she's off adventuring — trying anything from skiing in New England to scuba diving in Belize. Jeanne lives and parades in New Orleans with her husband, Jesse, and their dog and cats.

# THANK YOU

Thank you for reading *I Just Want to Be ME Again!* I'm delighted to be sharing this information with you. I hope you've found information here that helps you understand the journey that you're on and the changes that are happening to your body.

Throughout the book, I've told you about more information that's available on my website and I've collected all those references on one page: www.menopause.guru/book-resources.

I've also created a special course for you, the reader of this book, called Reveal the Roadblock. In this course, you'll have a chance to relax, listen to the messages your body has for you, and create your own plan to reach Midlife Nirvana. It contains video and audio descriptions of the exercises and a downloadable workbook to capture your answers and help you develop your plan. The course is based on the work described in Chapter Eight, and it's yours, free, just for the asking. You can get it at www.menopause.guru/rtr.

I also invite you to connect with me on Facebook. I'd love to answer your questions and help you with your plan!

*Website*: www.menopause.guru
*Facebook*: www.facebook.com/menopauseguru

## OTHER BOOKS BY JEANNE ANDRUS

*Lighten Up! A Game Plan for Losing Weight for Women in Menopause*, March, 2016

*Chill Out! How to Handle Hot Flashes and Other Annoying Symptoms of Menopause*, coming September, 2016

difference press

Difference Press offers entrepreneurs, including life coaches, healers, consultants, and community leaders, a comprehensive solution to get their books written, published, and promoted. A boutique-style alternative to self-publishing, Difference Press boasts a fair and easy-to-understand profit structure, low-priced author copies, and author-friendly contract terms. Its founder, Dr. Angela Lauria, has been bringing to life the literary ventures of hundreds of authors-in-transformation since 1994.

---

LET'S MAKE A DIFFERENCE WITH YOUR BOOK

You've seen other people make a difference with a book. Now it's your turn. If you are ready to stop watching and start taking massive action, reach out.

"Yes, I'm ready!"

In a market where hundreds of thousands books are published every year and are never heard from again, all participants of The Author Incubator have bestsellers that are actively changing lives and making a difference.

In two years we've created over 134 bestselling books in a row, 90% from first-time authors. We do this by selecting the highest quality and highest potential applicants for our future programs.

Our program doesn't just teach you how to write a book—our team of coaches, developmental editors, copy editors, art directors, and marketing experts incubate you from book idea to published bestseller, ensuring that the book you create can actually make a difference in the world. Then we give you the training you need to use your book to make the difference you want to make in the world, or to create a business out of serving your readers. If you have life-or world-changing ideas or services, a servant's heart, and the willingness to do what it REALLY takes to make a difference in the world with your book, go to http://theauthorincubator.com/apply/ to complete an application for the program today.

# OTHER BOOKS BY DIFFERENCE PRESS

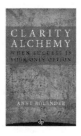

*Clarity Alchemy: When Success Is Your Only Option*

by Ann Bolender

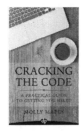

*Cracking the Code: A Practical Guide to Getting You Hired*

by Molly Mapes

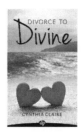

*Divorce to Divine: Becoming the Fabulous Person You Were Intended to Be*

by Cynthia Claire

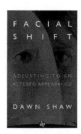

*Facial Shift: Adjusting to an Altered Appearance*

by Dawn Shaw

*Finding Clarity: Design a Business You Love and Simplify Your Marketing*

by Amanda H. Young

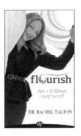

*Flourish: Have It All Without Losing Yourself*

by Dr. Rachel Talton

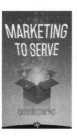

*Marketing To Serve: The Entrepreneur's Guide to Marketing to Your Ideal Client and Making Money with Heart and Authenticity*

by Cassie Parks

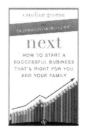

*NEXT: How to Start a Successful Business That's Right for You and Your Family*

by Caroline Greene

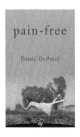

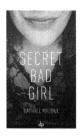

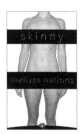

Pain Free: How I
Released 43 Years
of Chronic Pain

by Dottie DuParcé
(Author), John F.
Barnes (Foreword)

Secret Bad Girl:
A Sexual Trauma
Memoir and
Resolution Guide

by Rachael
Maddox

Skinny: The Teen
Girl's Guide to
Making Choices,
Getting the Thin
Body You Want,
and Having the
Confidence You've
Always Dreamed Of

by Melissa Nations

The Aging Boomers:
Answers to Critical
Questions for You,
Your Parents and
Loved Ones

by Frank M. Samson

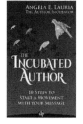

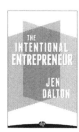

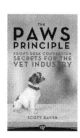

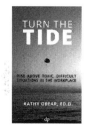

The Incubated
Author: 10 Steps to
Start a Movement
with Your Message

by Angela Lauria

The Intentional
Entrepreneur: How
to Be a Noisebreaker,
Not a Noisemaker

by Jen Dalton
(Author), Jeanine
Warisse Turner
(Foreword)

The Paws Principle:
Front Desk
Conversion Secrets
for the Vet Industry

by Scott Baker

Turn the Tide:
Rise Above Toxic,
Difficult Situations
in the Workplace

by Kathy Obear

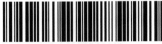

42483238R00093

Made in the USA
Middletown, DE
12 April 2017